"Devouring this book is a mercy-drenching, living-water experience. Eva reminds us of how God loves his girls by delighting in our womanhood and our need for rest, comfort, and safety. Throw on your bathrobe, put your feet up, and let these chapters zap the weariness from your journey. Thank you, Eva!"

Bonnie Keen, author, recording artist, speaker

"In this unique book, author Eva Marie Everson conveys a refreshing perspective: when women take care of their bodies (health, beauty, fashion, etc.) they are also taking care of their souls. After all, God made us in his image! Inspiring Scriptures and down-to-earth quotes from many of today's well-known women make this a volume of practical and spiritual help you won't want to miss. Buy one for a friend too!"

Karen O'Connor, author, *The Beauty of Aging*

"I love this book! Eva Marie is honest, funny, and practical and has an unusual ability to see right into the heart and mind of women—she comes right to our front door, gently steps in as a friend, and brings words of hope and wisdom we've been longing to hear. I have not yet met a woman to whom this book does not apply. I highly recommend this book—it's great for individual women, and it's fabulous for group study!"

Jennifer Rothschild, author, *Lessons I Learned in the Dark* and *Lessons I Learned in the Light*

"For the woman who wants to be beautiful, inside and out, Eva Marie has blended a refreshing tonic of wisdom and wit, biblical and practical insight for every woman's soul. Drink from this wonderful fountain, and you'll say 'ahhhh'!"

Patricia Raybon, author, *I Told the Mountain to Move*

"A book to revitalize you, body and soul! Like a refreshing trip to the spa, Eva Marie's book helps women realize that it's 'OK' to take care of ourselves, gives practical tools to help us do that, and—best of all—reminds us that we truly *are* beautiful . . . simply because we belong to God."

Nancy Stafford, actress; speaker; author, *Beauty by the Book* and *The Wonder of His Love*

"*Oasis* provides a retreat for women wishing to renew and revive themselves both in body and spirit. This spring of fresh water soothes the soul and provides a source of instruction for meeting all of your beauty needs on a practical level and emphasizing the importance of making God our wellspring."

Jill Krieger Swanson, image stylist, author

"*Oasis* illustrates the Scripture 'Man looks on the outward appearance, but God looks on the heart.' This book covers it all, from manicures and makeup to prayer and praise. During my years as an international Ford fashion model, I pursued outer beauty. Now, as a pastor's wife, I desire inner beauty too. *Oasis* provides the secret to finding a balance between the two and is full of valuable tips on being beautiful—inside and out."

Tonya Ruiz, former international Ford fashion model; author,
Beauty Quest: A Model's Journey

"Many thanks to Eva Marie Everson for offering both practical and inspirational tips on balancing body and soul. This is a difficult dance for all women, and I know *Oasis* will be an encouragement for the journey."

Lucinda Secrest McDowell, author,
Spa for the Soul: Rejuvenate Your Inner Life

"Filled with practical wisdom, inspiring stories, and faithful words, this book is the perfect recipe for beautiful living—inside and out."

Sharon Hanby-Robie, author, speaker, interior designer

"At last—a sensible look at merging the body beautiful with the body spiritual! Eva Marie's ability to focus on true inner beauty while encouraging healthy (and fun!) attention on pampering our femininity is completely refreshing."

Allison Bottke, author, *A Stitch in Time*;
founder, God Allows U-Turns

OASIS

a spa for body and soul

EVA MARIE EVERSON

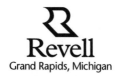

Revell
Grand Rapids, Michigan

© 2007 by Eva Marie Everson

Published by Fleming H. Revell
a division of Baker Publishing Group
P.O. Box 6287, Grand Rapids, MI 49516-6287
www.revellbooks.com

Printed in the United States of America

Library of Congress Cataloging-in-Publication Data
Everson, Eva Marie.
    Oasis : a spa for body and soul / Eva Marie Everson.
      p. cm.
    Includes bibliographical references (p.   ).
    ISBN 10: 0-8007-3134-4 (pbk.)
    ISBN 978-0-8007-3134-2 (pbk.)
    1. Beauty, Personal. 2. Health resorts. 3. Women—Health and hygiene.
  I. Title.
  RA778.E944 2007
  613′.12—dc22   2006033108

Unless otherwise indicated, Scripture is taken from the HOLY BIBLE, NEW INTERNATIONAL VERSION®. NIV®. Copyright © 1973, 1978, 1984 by International Bible Society. Used by permission of Zondervan. All rights reserved.

Scripture marked NASB is taken from the New American Standard Bible®, Copyright © 1960, 1962, 1963, 1968, 1971, 1972, 1973, 1975, 1977, 1995 by The Lockman Foundation. Used by permission.

Scripture marked KJV is taken from the King James Version of the Bible.

To my mother,
the most beautiful woman
—both in body and spirit—
I've ever known!

CONTENTS

A Note from the Author

I find it completely fascinating that I've written a book on physical and spiritual beauty. Typically, when one finds a book about women's physical beauty, and it's been written by a woman, there's a photo of said woman on the cover, within the flaps of the dust jacket, or on the back of the book. The woman is gorgeous. She's most definitely a former prom or pageant queen. She owns some famous boutique or has been a model. At the very least, she has developed a makeup line proven to take years off the appearance of a woman's face or has discovered an exercise program guaranteed to lift the buns, or your money back.

I am none of those things. I am the girl who grew up with straggly, nondescript brown hair, big brown eyes hidden behind Coke-bottle eyeglasses, funny-looking teeth (even the braces didn't help entirely), pale but freckled skin, and absolutely no sense of style.

But I had dreams of being beautiful. And I had a desire to love God passionately. (I hope you feel the same way about this. We should all strive to love him more dearly than we did the day before. I'll stop now; I feel an old *Godspell* song coming on . . .)

What I'm trying to say in these few lines where I get to say whatever I want to say however I want to say it is that I am not a beauty queen. But, I am a beautiful woman, simply because *I am a woman*. Women are beautiful. We were created to be, and we are.

> [Woman] is the crescendo, the final, astonishing work of God. Woman. In one last flourish creation comes to a finish not with Adam, but with *Eve*. She is the Master's finishing touch.
>
> John and Stasi Eldredge, *Captivating*

But, even with that said, I must remind you that we women choose how to exercise that beauty. You may or may not use moisturizer, read up on the latest fashions, get your nails done, or exercise regularly. That is totally up to you. If you'd rather wear old and tattered blue jeans instead of a Kasper suit any day of the week, well, then, you go, girl! If you'd rather deal with wrinkles than schedule application time or budget your income for the latest in a long line of youth serums, that's your prerogative. It won't make you any less beautiful to the One who matters most. In fact, using the best moisturizer in the world has absolutely no effect on God's view of you. To him, you are beautiful through and through because you are a reflection of his love. Period.

But to be honest with you, if you fall within that category, then part of this book simply is not for you. Yet, that doesn't mean you won't want to keep reading. Heavens, no. Even if you couldn't care less about what some call "high maintenance" issues . . . well, you may want to go ahead and read about them anyway. It'll give you something to snicker over. You can call your best girlfriend and say, "Can you believe women actually spend their days worrying about stuff like this? Who are these women, anyway?" and that will be okay with me and the rest of us who do care about stuff like that.

But there's a part of this book that I implore you not to skip. The part that deals with spiritual beauty. This is an area we cannot be "Oh, who cares?" about.

Because *he* cares. Your spiritual beauty is of utmost importance to him.

I believe that when God created woman, some of his best work was recognized. Not because of her physical beauty but because of what was stirring within her. No matter what we look like on the outside, when we are beautiful on the inside, *we are beautiful*. And, by the same token, no amount of physical beauty can make an ugly inner spirit pretty. (And we've all known these women, haven't we? Gorgeous to look at, but nasty, nasty, nasty on the inside.)

As you read—whether alone or within the study groups I've imagined you in, whether you're grabbing a few minutes between rushing the kids to school and soccer practice or enjoying a coffee break at your workplace or taking the bus or train or curling up in a comfy chair with a cup of tea—my prayer for you is that you will desire to know the One who created beauty, the One who *is* beauty.

And, in knowing him, you will become more beautiful still.

1

The Body Beautiful

Charm is deceptive, and beauty fleeting; but a woman who fears the LORD is to be praised.

Proverbs 31:30

Apparently, I am a high-maintenance chick.

Now, I think it's important for you to know that I never in all my years of puffing and fluffing thought of myself as being high maintenance. Then recently, while my husband and I sat with a group of friends, someone mentioned a certain woman (who shall remain nameless). "High maintenance," they called her.

"How do you figure that?" I asked. Yes, she is pretty and takes great care to ensure that all her features are accented and highlighted to perfection. Yes, she wears the nicest clothes, always flattering to her statuesque figure. Yes, she drives only top-of-the-line cars, eats at all the best restaurants, wraps only name-brand watches around her slender wrist. But, I mean . . . other than *that*?

On the way home, I said to my husband, "I'm glad I'm not high maintenance."

Dennis's head whipped around. "Say that again; I don't think I heard you correctly the first time," he quipped.

My mouth fell open in protest. "What do you mean by that crack?"

"*You* aren't high maintenance?"

"No," I reiterated, pointing a shaped and manicured nail at him. "I most assuredly am not."

"Then no one is," he said, shaking his head.

I kept my perfectly lined and painted bottom lip in a pout until a few days later when the truth finally seeped in. Or, I should say, knocked me over.

I was taking a shower at the time. Overhead, the adjustable showerhead (the one I said I just couldn't take a shower without) pelted out water at just the right pressure and temperature. Beside me, on the window shelf and neatly lined up, were bottles of what my daughter refers to as "product": shampoo, conditioner, body scrub, face scrub, little brush for scrubbing, foot scrub, back scrubber, loofah sponge, shaving cream, razors, body wash (both scented and unscented). You name it, it's there.

I raised my recently waxed brows.

Hmmmm.

I finished my shower, pulled back the double shower curtain (with matching accessories found throughout the room), and reached for a towel. A thick, thirsty one, color-coded to the room's décor. I propped a pedicured foot onto the tub's marble ledge and began to pat myself dry (I learned a long time ago that a lady should never rub her skin) beginning with my feet and legs and working my way upward. Done, I wrapped my hair in the towel, reached for a drier one to wrap myself in, and stepped out . . .

And over to my vanity, where what my husband calls "Cosmetic City" awaited me.

Lotions—hand, face, feet, body—more scrubs, body sprays, perfumes, some seaweed extract proven (though not by me at this point) to reduce cellulite, and a $150 toothbrush guaranteed to beat away the plaque. Nearby, a candle graced the top of a golden pedestal, and I lit it. The CD player from the adjoining master suite entertained me with my favorite boudoir music of the week. I sat at the vanity, reaching for the first of many steps in becoming . . . oh my. High maintenance.

Okay, so it's true. I get my nails done and my hair trimmed on a regular basis, and I am passionate about jewelry. I can be talked into a shopping spree—even if only to window-shop—at any given moment, no matter what's going on in my life. I get up early in the morning, walk no less than two miles in the heat and humidity, go to bed rather late at night, and nap in the afternoons.

I wear makeup every single day, if only to impress my pets, but mostly to impress my husband—and on the off chance that someone comes to the door.

I like fine dining. My idea of roughing it is sleeping at the Ritz Carlton. I adore afternoon teas in cute little teahouses and won't drink coffee at dinner if it's not served in a cup and saucer.

Could there be a group for someone like me? I wondered, pondering myself in the vanity's mirror. *Hello, my name is Eva Marie Everson, and I'm a high-maintenance chick.*

For months I was plagued by this thought. Me, high maintenance. What did just those two words say about me as a woman . . . as a person . . . as a Christian?

My shower time became unbearable. All I could do (as I continued to use all those wonderful products) was think about my lifestyle. *It's "high maintenance," yes, but not as high maintenance as some of the women I know. And, if I use certain products, wear certain name brands, afford myself certain pleasures and pamperings, does that mean I'm less of a Christian than I thought?*

The more I wrestled with it, the more God began showing me certain truths.

Body wash . . . *Eva Marie, are you washed in the blood?*

Body lotion . . . *Eva Marie, do you care for your spiritual body?*

Leave-in hair conditioner . . . *Eva Marie, do you wrap yourself daily in my armor? Are you kept strong by the Holy Spirit?*

The latest fashion . . . *Eva Marie, are you clothed in righteousness?*

So, the question, then, is *not* whether or not I am high maintenance in my personal life but whether or not I'm high maintenance in my spiritual life. Am I a high-maintenance Christian chick?

The Body Beautiful—Physical

> I praise you because I am fearfully and wonderfully
> made;
> your works are wonderful, I know that full well.
>
> Psalm 139:14

She's a total package: long, shiny hair, a face that could launch a thousand ships, and a body that—even after giving birth to a houseful of children—could rival that of any high school cheerleader. Ask her what her secret is, and she'll tell you, "I work at it." The result of her hard work is a body that works *for* itself rather than *against* itself.

I understand the latter concept all too well. As a writer, I sit in a chair many hours a day. A few years ago, when I began working as a freelance writer, I was trim, in shape, and feeling pretty good about myself. Three years later I was staring in disbelief at the sadistic scales in my physician's office.

"Liar!" I screamed. But the truth of the matter was I'd gained thirty pounds over the course of a little more than two years.

It wasn't just my vanity that was in trouble. With my new "fluffy" middle, my back had taken a beating (my bones and joints aren't the best in the world anyway). I couldn't quite understand what one had to do with the other until my doctor explained that the stomach muscles support the spine. Let one go, and the other crumbles.

So I decided to choose a diet plan and shed some unwanted pounds. Problem is, there are tons of plans out there, and few of them include chocolate, without which no day is complete. This could only mean one thing: diet . . . not dieting. *Dieting* is depriving myself, feeling hungry and miserable. I know. I've tried dieting my whole adult life. *Diet* is filling my body with healthy choices from the basic food groups, not denying myself all my favorite foods and then crumbling into an emotional heap when I "fall."

Next, I picked an exercise program. Again, scores of them out there. Should I go to a gym and work out with others? Should I sink tons of money into a home gym or should I simply buy myself a Walkman and trek around the block several times a day while listening to praise tunes?

Should I jog? (Quick answer: no.)

What about something fun like ballroom dancing? I proposed the possibility to my dear husband, who laughed out loud and then resolutely said, "Not gonna happen."

Swimming? I love swimming. I used to be on a swim team way back when I was but a child. I performed water ballet. I don't have a pool in my backyard, but my homeowner's association dues afford me the joys of using the neighborhood pool—along with about a dozen or so children and a few loud and obnoxious adults. Not to mention the P-Y-Ts (Pretty Young Things) wearing their P-P-Ss (Pretty Petite Suits). So, swimming as an exercise plan was O-U-T.

Stair-climbing versus taking the elevator? Yeah, that would be good, if I had a flight of stairs or an elevator in my house.

So, I chose walking, one of the finest, most beneficial exercises known to humanity. No expensive equipment necessary other than a good pair of walking shoes and maybe a Walkman or some other device designed for sending out music.

When it comes to physical beauty, Michelle McKinney Hammond, author of *The Diva Principle*, says, "A trip to an art museum always reminds me that besides being a temple of the Holy Spirit, my body is a work of art! My advice is to take good care of your body—no matter what size you are. The better you feel, the better you will look. Nurture your skin with moisturizing gels and creams. (My favorite is Amazing Grace by Philosophy and Ambre Extreme or Musk by Kiehl's.) Smell good and don't hide under layers that don't enhance your best attributes. The bottom line? The more you celebrate the skin you're in, the more you'll be admired by others. Confidence is the greatest beauty secret I know!"

I also decided to drink water—lots and lots of it—every day. Water is a wonderful secret to overall fitness. In fact, a body's survival depends on water, and water has been ranked by experts as right up there with oxygen when it comes to life's essentials. It carries the food nutrients to the body's cells and cushions joints, protecting them even from the shock of exercise.

The result? I'm currently down two dress sizes and working toward more.

The Body Beautiful—Spiritual

> Do you not know that your body is a temple of the Holy Spirit, who is in you, whom you have received from God?
>
> 1 Corinthians 6:19

Just as it is important that we take care of our physical bodies, so it is important that we take care of our spiritual selves. In 1 Corinthians 12:12–27, Paul expands on the theme of physical body compared to spiritual body. We are, he writes, the body of Christ. What is done to the body is done to Christ himself.

The connection between the physical body and the spiritual body does not begin in the New Testament, however. Old Testament writers were just as knowledgeable of the parallel. When man first sinned—a spiritual act—both the spiritual and the physical body were affected. Spiritually, our eternal lives were now at stake. Physically, man would "till the soil" and woman would "give birth in pain." Physical, spiritual, and emotional wounds were now capable of slicing into us. While on this earth we would forever be required as a race to take care of ourselves in every area of our lives.

Just as the physical body needs a proper diet, so does the spiritual. Without a balance of the Word, prayer, and fellowship, we cannot grow. These three are the diet, exercise, and water that make up our spiritual needs.

The Word

Joshua 1:8 reads: "Do not let this Book of the Law depart from your mouth; meditate on it day and night, so that you may be careful to do everything written in it. Then you will be prosperous and successful." This is the Lord God Almighty instructing his servant Joshua before the greatest challenge of his life: he is about to cross over into the enemy-inhabited Promised Land and must conquer it. The Lord's instruction to be "strong and courageous" (vv. 6, 7, 9) depends on Joshua's time spent in the Word.

Prayer

Paul wrote, "Do not be anxious about anything, but in everything, by prayer and petition, with thanksgiving, present your requests to God" (Phil. 4:6). Paul wrote much on prayer, reminding us of what a precious gift it is, instructing us to pray "continuously." Naturally it is not possible to remain in our prayer closets without ever coming out, but we are to take on an attitude of prayer. This requires an understanding that prayer is more than our running into the throne room and barking out orders to God. Prayer is our being in a constant state of understanding that we are in his presence, talking with him as we would a friend—a father—and being ever intent on hearing his voice as he speaks to us.

Fellowship

The second chapter of Acts impresses on us the importance of fellowship when it comes to growing both the individual body as well as the church body. Being with one another is a dress rehearsal for heaven, in my way of thinking.

Recently, as I walked around Glorieta, New Mexico (a LifeWay Conference Center), with several hundred other Christians, I got a sense of heaven. The constant fellowship, the talking about God with words of praise and adoration, the sitting together in a little coffee shop and exchanging our personal love stories about the Savior. I felt reenergized! Excited and blessed beyond belief to be a part of this heavenly body!

Questions for Personal Reflection or Group Study

1. What is your favorite form of physical exercise, and how often do you do it?
2. Do you consider yourself "high maintenance" where your physical body is concerned? Define what you mean.
3. Are you "high maintenance" in your spiritual walk? Define what you mean.

When it comes to spiritual beauty, author and Women of Faith speaker Patsy Clairmont says, "I stay spiritually beautiful by purposing to keep my cantankerous mind full of God's life-giving Word. 'Thy words were found, and I did eat them; and thy word was unto me the joy and rejoicing of mine heart'" (Jer. 15:16 KJV).

4. Water makes up two-thirds of your body's weight and is one of the most important factors in staying healthy. Jesus referred to himself as the Living Water, saying, "Everyone who drinks this water will be thirsty again, but whoever drinks the water I give him will never thirst. Indeed, the water I give him will become in him a spring of water welling up to eternal life" (John 4:13–14). How much physical water do you drink a day? How much of the Living Water do you drink a day?

Here's a Valuable Tip

You don't have to be rich to afford good beauty products, and—if you are financially comfortable—you don't have to spend all your money to feel pretty. Actually, there are three categories of women out there when it comes to purchasing beauty products.

1. Money's Tight
2. Money Conscious
3. Money's No Object

Whatever category you fall into, you *can* afford to take care of yourself. For example, when it comes to most products—and if you are in the first category—head on over to your favorite drugstore or discount store such as Wal-Mart, K-Mart, Target, etc. You can go to Drugstores.com and find a host of products at very reasonable prices. There's always Avon and Mary Kay as well, though some of their products fall more in line with the second category.

Money-Conscious Women might be more apt to head over to Body Works, the Body Shop, L'Occitane, Crabtree and Evelyn . . . these are but a few of the specialty stores you can find out there in malls, strip malls, airports, or streets designed just for shoppers. Money's No Object Women shop at a variety of department stores, specialty stores, spas, etc. But it doesn't necessarily mean these products will be any better than the ones the Money's Tight Women are purchasing at Walgreen's.

And, you don't always have to go to expensive salons and spas. If you have a training school in your area, you can find tomorrow's professionals working at a fraction of the cost.

Finally (and while we are talking money), make sure there is as much a balance in your personal pampering as in your monetary stewardship. The woman who gives before she receives is truly the most blessed of all.

2

BATH AND SHOWER PRODUCTS

I bathed you with water and . . . put ointments on you.

Ezekiel 16:9

If you have made it this far in the book, perhaps you've asked yourself some fairly important questions, such as, "Am I as high maintenance in my spiritual life as in my physical life? Do I spend as much time daily on my spiritual self as I do on my physical self?" Or, if you don't spend a whole lot of time on your physical self, the important question is "Do I spend adequate time on my spiritual self?"

I hope—no, I pray—that you've not come down on yourself too much. That's beating yourself up, something high-maintenance, low-maintenance, and no-maintenance chicks should never do. Recognizing your weak areas is important, yes. But beating yourself up is a no-no.

For example, I have confessed that my weakest muscles (or set of muscles) are the ones around my middle. For me, the first step to working on my six-pack abs (I'm up to about a one-pack) is recognizing the weakness and the outcome of the weakness. Remember? I said my back had suffered.

See? I confessed, but I have yet to beat myself up (though a few times I have wept over my inability to say no to chocolate).

I also confessed to being high maintenance—something I had never considered until my husband pointed it out, leading me to recognize all the little things I do to take care of myself. The more I saw high maintenance in my physical self—beginning with my shower products—the more I wondered about how much time I spent taking care of my spiritual self. I pose the same question for you as well.

So, with this chapter, let's look at the one common thing we women do—(typically) every day—in order to take care of our physical selves. Let's look at "the bath."

The Body Beautiful—Physical

> Wash and perfume yourself, and put on your best clothes.
>
> Ruth 3:3

Tell my granddaughter that it's time to take a bath, and she jumps up from whatever she may be doing, runs down the hall, and begins stripping out of her clothes. Bath time is fun time! Warm water cascades from the faucet and—with the help of some bubble bath—a river of soapy froth is formed. Her colorful alphabet bath toys (still there from a previous bath) float almost joyfully, anticipating the little cutie who will slip into the water and play for the better part of the next half hour. Sometimes her bath is only for the fun of it; other times it's an absolute necessity.

Bathing, in our American culture, is a daily ritual designed to wash away the day's dirt and body odor. Sometimes a bath or shower is not for the purpose of cleansing but for the purpose of relaxation or mental renewal. "All I want to do is take a hot shower and go to bed" isn't usually said because we're dirty but because we're tired or in need of stress relief.

Modern bathrooms often have both shower and tub. Some tubs are lined with jets for pulsating water toward tense muscles. But the bath was not always as we know it today. For example, we know from Exodus 2:5 that Pharaoh's daughter went down to the river to bathe. (Aren't you shy ladies glad you weren't a part of those times?)

Many times, for God's people in the ancient Middle East, bathing was for the purpose of becoming ceremonially clean. The Romans installed lavish "public baths" where citizens could exercise, bathe, and socialize. And there was a time when Europeans feared the bath—both nobility and commoners rarely washed but rather applied talcum powder. (Glad I didn't live back then, either . . .)

Today we have entire stores dedicated to the art of bathing, where one can buy bath oils, gels, salts, bubble baths, and specialty soaps (made with extracts of herbs, fruits, and vegetables, vitamins E and C, etc.). They come in a vari-

> Bonnie Watkins, a high school teacher from Austin, Texas, says, "When it comes to baths, the more bubbles and candles, the better. My favorites are candles from Yankee Candle (lemon lime and pear) and bath products from Bath & Body Works (plumeria, because my beloved prodigal son was the first to give it to me, and when I smell it I am reminded to pray for him). I always light the candle fifteen minutes before I take my bath."

**PRODUCTS NOT
TO OVERLOOK**

Skin Towels
Sponges
Bath Gloves
Bath Pillows
Body Brushes
Body Buffers
Loofah Sponges

ety of scents designed to relax, stimulate, or even put you in a romantic mood. Consumers can choose to leave their bath smelling like flowers or fruit and just about everything in between.

Turning Your Bath into a Personal Spa

Very few of us can afford to go to a spa on a daily basis, and you don't have to. Your own bathroom can become a personal oasis for you if you follow a few simple steps.

1. Turn off distractions. Unplug the phone. Shut the door. (If you are a mother with small children, certainly do not do this unless you have another adult or older child in charge of the little ones.)
2. Light a few candles. You don't have to invest your life's savings, either. Head down to your favorite dollar store and grab a few scented candles for a dollar each. They smell wonderful and burn for a long time.
3. Add some music. (But don't put a radio or any electric device near your bathwater. Please!) Be sure you don't rock the house, either. Something soothing and uplifting playing quietly in the background is best.
4. If you are showering, take your time. If you can, purchase a massage head for your shower. If not, begin with a nice warm spray and, when you are done with your shower, turn the water to cool for the final rinse. You'll feel wonderful!

5. If you are relaxing in the tub, grab a book or magazine and an inflatable pillow. But, try not to go to sleep!

The Body Beautiful—Spiritual

> Cleanse me with hyssop, and I will be clean;
> wash me, and I will be whiter than snow.
>
> Psalm 51:7

There is a popular song on Christian charts in which the singer states that he's "been to the water and come out clean." Like physical bathing, spiritual bathing takes on many purposes; namely, being baptized, daily cleansing from the world's impurities, and being washed by God in a sort of disciplinary action.

Before beginning his earthly ministry, Jesus went down to the Jordan River, where John the Baptist was baptizing those who heard his message of redemption—of turning from

When it comes to a luxurious bubble bath, speaker and author of *A Stitch in Time*, Allison Bottke, says, "You can never have too many bubbles. I buy bubble bath in gallon jugs from Wal-Mart—no kidding—and pour oodles of it directly under the faucet. Disappearing under mounds of bubbles sends me back to a time when I was a little girl without a care in the world. It's a good feeling. Aside from bubble bath, when it comes to body soaps and skin lotions, I'm addicted to anything from L'Occitane. Their almond shower oil smells scrumptious, and all the lotions leave your skin feeling like silk. It's pricey stuff, but hey, I save on bubble bath and splurge on lotion!"

the old self and back toward God. Jesus' request to John to be baptized by him shocked the young evangelist. "I need to be baptized by you, and do you come to me?" John said to Jesus. How could John—who was sinful man—possibly "cleanse" one who was without sin? Jesus insisted, stating that it "fulfilled all righteousness." As Jesus came up out of the water—dripping, his clothes no doubt clinging to him—the Spirit of God came down as a dove and perched upon him, and the Father's voice declared his pleasure at what the Son had done. Jesus' obedience to the ritual of baptism brought about joyous declaration from the Trinity, in revelation to the people.

Rejuvenated for the task ahead, Jesus headed out into the desert . . . and toward bringing about salvation for humankind.

I walk in the mornings. Here in Florida, that bit of exercise takes on a whole new meaning in the summer months. I can barely stand being with myself as I head home in my car from the area where I walk. If my husband is still home upon my arrival, I state, "Don't come near me. I stinketh!" A good shower later and I am, once again, presentable.

Though we are not baptized by water on a daily basis, each and every day affords us the opportunity to be bathed in the blood of the Lamb, to be purified from our sins—which cause us to stinketh—so that we may draw close to the Father.

David's cry to be "washed with hyssop" is more accurately read "purge me with hyssop." David had sinned big-time and was in need of a cleansing that would wash away not only those stains that were obvious but also the ones that had bled down into his very soul. He had separated himself from the love of his life, the Lord.

Jill Eileen Smith, a piano teacher from Sterling Heights, Michigan, says, "I shower—not a big bathtub fan—but I love Aveda's Rosemary Mint body wash. The scent is not overpowering, yet it seems to wake me up. I come away from the shower feeling not only clean but refreshed."

There are times when we, like David, allow ourselves to slip into fleshly desire and out of the will of God. We know we've done wrong, and we keep our eyes downcast. Knowing God is just behind us, we dare not look over our shoulders lest we catch the look in his eye. Our hearts are nearly empty of joy. As day drags into endless day, we become more encrusted with our own filth. We can sprinkle ourselves with all the talcum in the world, and we'll still be rank. It isn't until we submit to a washing from God—a true scrubbing away of the old skin cells—that we can be presentable again.

The washing is easy; it is. We, like David, need only to cry out to the Lord to wash us clean. The blood of Jesus will symbolically wash over us, making us clean in the eyes of God. And then our spiritual bodies are as clean as the day we were born. With this cleansing we can walk out to perform our daily ministry.

Questions for Personal Reflection or Group Study

1. Where and how were you baptized?
2. If you were of an age at the time in which you can remember your baptism, how did you feel afterward? Be specific.
3. Do you daily ask God to cleanse you of your sins, or only when you know you've sinned "big-time"?

4. Define "purge." How does that differ from mere "washing"?
5. Have you ever felt completely isolated from the Lord? What happened to drive you away? What happened to bring you back?

Here's a Valuable Tip

When it comes to purchasing items for your bath, go online. Drugstores.com is an excellent place to find your bath products or any of the others I'll mention in this book. Or, you can go to the websites of the specialty stores such as Bath & Body Works and department stores such as Macy's and Neiman Marcus. If you've got a computer and a credit card, the world of bath products is your oyster!

3

Naptime, Bedtime, and Time Away

The LORD replied, "My Presence will go with you, and I
will give you rest."

Exodus 33:14

I grew up near the coast of Georgia. Heading for the water—
whether a lake, a stream, a river, or the ocean—was as much
a part of my life as breathing. Many of our family members
and friends owned the "house at the coast" or the "getaway
at the beach." Some were little cabins; others were something
akin to a condo. But they all had the rich and intoxicating
scent of sand, water, heat, and fish. That may not sound
rich and intoxicating to you, but if you grew up near the
water, you understand.

As a teenager, I spent countless hours heading toward
the sand and surf of Tybee Island just outside of Savannah.
Days of bodysurfing, lying out on beach towels under the
blistering sun, and smelling like sweat, salt, and coconut
or baby oil come to mind as easily as yesterday's dinner. I

can lick my lips and taste the ocean, even now. I can close my eyes and breathe the salty air, hear the tide pounding against the shore. For me, the seashore is like a little piece of heaven, and it continues to beckon me toward it. "Come back, come back," it calls, the voice of it fading in the breeze. "Come back and rest, relax, play. Come back to the days when you had energy to burn and time to spare. Come back."

Today I live in Florida. I'm less than an hour's drive from the shoreline. Whenever I go, I vow I won't wait so long to go again. Then life has its way, and months go by and I haven't returned. But at least twice a year, I find myself sitting in a beach chair with a good book in one hand and a cold drink in the other. While seagulls squawk over my head, dipping and diving as they search for food (or a handout from my pretzel bag), I look up and out over the ocean, toward the horizon, and wonder, *How magnificent is my God!*

Let me give you a clue about high-maintenance chicks: we get away. Whether for fifteen minutes, an afternoon, a day, or a weekend, we get *away*! Not just because we deserve

Michelle Griep, a homeschooling mom and freelance writer from St. Louis Park, Minnesota, says, "I nap every day I possibly can (twenty to thirty minutes). Naptime is my all-time favorite time. When my kids were little, that was their 'independent reading' time. Naptime is my recharge time. My day is spent giving, giving, giving to everyone, and that's my short time away for me. And, usually by about two in the afternoon, I'm starting to drag physically, so with a little rest, I can be the Energizer Bunny for the rest of the day."

it but also because our bodies need it. We need it like the water and the air we cannot live without.

The Body Beautiful—Physical

> This is the resting place, let the weary rest . . . This is the place of repose.
>
> Isaiah 28:12

What is it about a nap that makes us fight to keep from taking one when we are young? Yet, as adults, the thought of a little siesta in the afternoons sounds like manna in the desert. Why is that, exactly?

A year ago I was visiting a friend for several days in her mountain home. We sat in her living room one midafternoon, having put in quite a busy morning and early afternoon. Curled up on the sofa and feeling tired but happy, I was just about to suggest a nice cup of coffee when suddenly she said, "I'm going to take a little nap. See you in fifteen minutes."

And with that, she stretched out in her recliner, closed her eyes, and was out. I'm talking O-U-T! I watched in total

THREAD COUNT

If you want a good night's sleep, begin with the purchase of good bed linens. Thread count (the number of threads per square inch of fabric) is what you're looking for. High-quality sheets have a thread count of at least 180, but that doesn't necessarily mean 180 is the best. Thread count of 200–220 is good quality, but 230–280 is better, and 300–400 is the best. You can even get thread count up to 1000 these days, but my sources tell me that anything over 500 is a waste of good money. While looking at thread count, you'll also want to note the yarn size of your sheets. High yarn sizes indicate the finer yarns and cotton of the highest quality.

amazement and then closed my own eyes for a few minutes of repose. I felt myself slipping into la-la land, my shoulders relaxing, and the nerves in my body twitching a bit here and there. I laid my head over to a small pillow and began to drool. (I'm just so sure I did!)

Then, *bam!* I heard the recliner return to its upright position and my friend spring out of it. I jumped, sitting straight up, blinking in the light until her face became clear again. She was grinning like a cat.

"Ah," she said. "That was a nice nap."

I looked down at my watch. Exactly fifteen minutes had passed since she'd closed her eyes. "How'd you do that?" I asked, amazed.

"I don't know," she said. "I've just trained my body to accept the fifteen-minute nap. Now I can do another half a day's work!"

The Importance of the Nap

We all know that naps are important for children. They're growing, and they need that downtime in order to do so properly. (They're also cranky as all get-out if they don't get enough sleep!) Adults need naps too. (We're growing as well, but in our case we're growing *older*.)

Some cultures have learned both the beauty and importance of a nap. It's called *"siesta."*

Years ago, the siesta period would last as long as three hours, beginning at about noon or one o'clock, though today it may last only a couple of hours.

A couple of hours? Amazing. Shops close down. People go home and crawl between the covers or gather on verandas and in little courtyards to sip on drinks and chat a bit before lowering their lashes and snoozing a while. Can you imagine what might happen to the American way of life if we all stopped doing what we do, buzzing around like bees intent on drawing nectar from every single flower in the garden, and just rested a bit? In the American way of thinking, everything we know about our workdays would go flush down the toilet, but in reality, we'd get so much more done. In reality, we're never going to get it all done anyway, so we may as well nap!

I have a friend, a British chap, who lives in the Atlanta area. One day my daughter and I drove nearly eight hours for a visit with him and his family. As soon as we arrived at the house—at about three o'clock in the afternoon—he helped us settle in our room and then headed upstairs; I thought he was going to retrieve something. After a good half hour with not a single sound or a muffled footstep coming from above our heads, I crept up the staircase, peeked around the corner of a wall, looked into the library, and found my friend napping on the sofa. I later learned this was a part of his daily ritual and had been for as long as he could remember. He can do twice as much *with* the nap as *without*.

Considerable studies have been done (even by the United States Army) that prove the importance of the nap (though some like to refer to it as a "break"). Taking some time away from your work (or whatever it is you do during the day) helps to relieve stress and irritability, adds mental focus, and leads to a decrease in "human error," which is most often due to fatigue.

Did you know that many creative people get their best ideas right after a nap or a walk (to clear the cobwebs), or just as they are waking from sleep? It's true. As a creative person, I can wholeheartedly say it's true!

For example, the very first book I ever wrote was "birthed" during a morning walk. And, once when I was trying to figure out how to make an upcoming speech inspirational and exciting, and after I'd exhausted every idea I could think of, I laid down for twenty minutes with some nice, soft music and closed my eyes. Ten minutes into my rest, the idea for what is now my most popular speaking topic was born.

You'll read differing opinions about how long a nap should last. Some say ten minutes will do the body good, others say twenty. Nearly all say that more than a half hour is too much.

Whether you take ten, fifteen, or twenty minutes, you might want to observe the following tips for making the nap all the more sweet.

- Find a favorite spot. Maybe it's the sofa in your family room or love seat in your sitting room. Maybe it's your bed. Crawl under the sheets or lay on top of the covers. As long as you're happy!
- Make sure your pillow is comfy. What's the point of a nap if you're going to wake up with a stiff neck?
- If you work outside of your home during the day, find a safe, quiet place for napping. Perhaps you can drive your car to a park, lake, etc. Or, go to an out-of-the-way room somewhere in your office building.
- If you are at home, be sure to lock your doors. If you are often bothered by knocks on the door or the ringing of the doorbell, put a little sign out.
- Take the phone off the hook. Whatever "emergency" might occur can wait fifteen minutes.

Sleep Time

Most people today complain of not getting enough sleep. "Early to bed, early to rise" is no longer observed. Thanks in part to alarm clocks, we drag ourselves from the comfort of our covers way before the sun peeks its rays over the horizon.

In the dark of early morning, we shuffle into the kitchen to make a pot of coffee or to brew a cup of caffeinated tea. How else can we possibly make it till midmorning? Shoulders humped, we begin our morning rituals. Sometimes that means adding another load of laundry to the washing machine. Or, turning on our computers to check our email while the coffee perks. Or, curling up with the news so we can find out how bad it is out there, reminding ourselves once again that we'd have been better off keeping the covers pulled over our heads.

Such is life.

Nighttime is no better. Thanks in part to that cup of coffee we had at three or four in the afternoon so we could make it till dinnertime (or the one we had with dinner so we could make it till bedtime), or the two-hour television special that started at nine, or the myriad of activities we schedule for the evening, we don't fall into bed until eleven. Or, for some of us—myself included—until after midnight.

Nope, we don't get enough of the old shut-eye. But what I wrote above is only part of the culprit. Many people today find themselves sleeping in bedrooms that are used for everything and anything other than sleeping. This is the room where bills are paid, meals are eaten, or television is watched. Some people even keep their exercise equipment in their bedroom (for hanging towels and discarded clothes on, don't you know).

Bedrooms should be about sleeping, not about bill paying, exercising, and the like. Call it high maintenance if you want to, but we need our eight hours of sleep!

Though some of us can get away with seven hours, humans—as a whole—do best with what is considered average: seven to eight hours. This is because of the amount of time needed to get through sleep cycles, which I'll explain in a minute. First, let's look at what sleep actually is.

Sleep is the natural periodic suspension of consciousness during which the powers of the body are restored.[1]

"Suspension of consciousness." I like that.

Here's what I *don't* like about sleep: we aren't awake to enjoy it.

Recently I spent the night with my daughter (she was sick, and, although an adult, she needed her mommy). Jessica has the most fabulous bed. Fluffy pillows, pillow-top mattress, five-hundred-thread-count linens, and a down duvet. "Mercy's sake, Jessica. If I were you, I'd never leave this bed." It was pure heaven, I tell you. "Only problem is, once you're asleep, how are you to enjoy it? If I were you, I'd eat here, watch TV here, talk on the phone here. If I didn't have to get up, I never would."

Sleep, glorious sleep. It comes in five stages, and those five stages are repeated several times during the night. Here's the breakdown:

Stage One: "Sleepy Time." Though every so often the proverbial "as soon as my head hits the pillow" may happen, typically we slip in and out of a state of drowsiness before we actually go to sleep. Our muscles begin to relax, and our eyes move behind closed lids ever so slowly. This is the time when it's easiest to be awakened (which would lead to, "Ugh! I just fell asleep"). Stage one typically takes about five to ten minutes.

Stage Two: "Deeper Still." Though this is not deep sleep, we've now moved from stage one (drowsiness) to stage two (light sleep). As our heart rate slows down, our body temp decreases. (Though most menopausal women would argue that at no time during the night does our body temperature ever decrease.) Eye movement stops and brain waves slow down. Fifty percent of your sleep cycle is spent in stage two.

Stages Three and Four: "The Deepest Part." During these two deep sleep stages, there is no eye movement or muscle activity. This is the part of sleep where, if you are suddenly awakened, it takes several minutes to get your heart rate back to normal and get yourself acclimated to the world as you know it.

Stage Five: "REM—Rapid Eye Movement." REM typically occurs about an hour and a half after falling asleep. During REM, breathing becomes shallow, irregular, and rapid; eyes jerk back and forth and up and down; and the muscles in our arms and legs become temporarily paralyzed. Heart rate increases, blood pressure rises. This is where we dream. (And, if you're lucky, in color!)

Sleep cycles typically take about 90 to 110 minutes. The average person will go through the cycle four or five times a night, should they sleep for eight hours.

Lack of the proper amount of sleep can lead to a plethora of problems. Things like anxiousness, impatience, lack of concentration, difficulty in learning, difficulty in remembering, and—are you ready for this?—inability to "play well with others."

Far too many women are sleep deprived today. Their solution is to make up for it on weekends. This is not a good idea. The best thing you can do for yourself and your sleep health is to go to bed at the same time and get up at the same time every day of the week. And, of course, take naps if possible.

Getaways

Okay, so here's the thing about "getting away." If you pack a cell phone (okay, you can *pack* it, but for heaven's sake keep it turned off, other than in an emergency, and emergency being translated as "death"), laptop, or any other modern means of contact with the outside world, you haven't really gotten away. You've merely moved geographically.

A getaway can be anything from a trip to Starbucks or any other favorite coffee shop, bookstore, lake, hiking trail, etc., to a two-week cruise. But if you take work or anything that might compel you to work, you have quite simply failed in the whole getaway process.

I have a friend who is also a colleague. She and I can "see" each other online and have the capability of IM-ing anytime we'd like. And we often do. We ask questions about everything from work-related issues to what we're having for dinner.

Every so often one of us shoots an IM to the other that reads something like this: "I gotta go to Office Max. Ten minutes???"

Now, you have to know how to translate this little message. First, Office Max is right next door to Books-A-Million. Second, there is an awesome coffee shop, Joe Muggs, in Books-A-Million, complete with overstuffed couches and little round wooden tables. Third, Joe Muggs employees in this particular Books-A-Million make a mean latte. Fourth, their cake ain't half bad either, though neither my friend nor I will ever admit to eating it.

You see, the trip to Office Max is an excuse for leaving our desks, though we don't really need an excuse other than to say, "We need a getaway!"

A half hour of sitting in the comfy furniture, sipping a latte, laughing with my friend, perusing the book selections (and maybe even buying something) is just what I need to return to my home office and crank out more work.

Not everyone can just walk out of his or her workplace, though, and I understand that. But, perhaps you can allot yourself a few minutes of time, once a week, before or after work. Or, set aside one lunch hour a week for "yourself." This won't be about eating. This will be your little minivacation. Whatever it is you enjoy doing—taking a walk, going to a special café, reading a book, visiting a friend. You name it, you do it!

The Body Beautiful—Spiritual

> By the seventh day God had finished the work he had been doing; so on the seventh day he rested from all his work. And God blessed the seventh day and made it holy, because on it he rested from all the work of creating that he had done.
>
> Genesis 2:2–3

If I say "Susannah Wesley," will the name ring a bell? Probably so, if you're Methodist. Susannah Wesley was the mother of John and Charles Wesley, who were largely responsible for founding Meth-

You've no doubt heard about home party companies such as Tupperware, PartyLite, Mary Kay, and Premier Designs jewelry, but have you heard of Quiet Places? Quiet Places has three distinctive product lines that apply to the heart, the home, and the mind. Journals, devotional books, and Christian living books are offered to quiet the heart. Home accessories in conjunction with a full line of gourmet scented candles, potpourri, and room sprays are designed to make the home inviting. Bubble baths, lotions, and a relaxation CD calm a stressed mind. For more information, go to www .quietplacesforyou.com.

When it comes to naps, author (*The Potluck Club*) and speaker Linda Evans Shepherd says, "Ahhh, the nap—or shall I say, the pause that refreshes. No longer are naps just for the cranky, they're for those of us on 'crankiness prevention.' Also, I've discovered they are the perfect gift. Though a nap is not something you can buy, it's something you can do not only for yourself but for those who love you. I also find that a day with an afternoon nap means an evening with more energy and vitality. Taking a nap is less fattening than chocolate ice cream, it's cheaper than Starbucks, and it delivers the same amount of energy as all those calories and caffeine combined."

odism and who were a part of the era known as the Great Awakening.

Though she gave birth to nineteen children, only nine survived. Two of those children were deformed. For six hours every day, Susannah homeschooled her kids (and this was way before homeschooling became a popular form of education). But it is also written of her that when she sat down heavily in a chair and threw her apron over her head, the children knew she'd "gone away to be with God." It was time to leave Mama alone.

In other words, Susannah Wesley—with everything she had going on in her unmodernized life—took time away from the busyness of it all and prayed. It wasn't Joe Muggs at Books-A-Million or sitting on the shore of a great ocean, but it was the best she could do, and it was obviously important to her.

God—the tireless Creator of the universe—also rested.

Did you hear that? God rested. In fact, he found resting to be so important, he linked it to holiness. *Holiness.*

We also know that Jesus found "away" time to be important. When he had sanded his last piece of wood and chiseled his last bit of stone, he took a walk along the Jordan River, met his cousin John (the Baptizer), was baptized, and thus began his ministry, his calling as Messiah, to draw our hearts back to the heart of God. Before uttering one word of his message, before healing the sick, or raising the dead, or declaring the fulfillment of the Scriptures, Jesus went away to fast and pray.

Okay, so there was that temptation thing, but because of the time he'd spent in prayer with the Father—because of that communion and in spite of the fact that he was hungry and thirsty—Jesus was able to withstand the temptations of Satan. In the end, the angels came and tended to him. What a beautiful picture! Even more so to know that when we need time away—and when we make that time and allow ourselves to be immersed in God's rest and holiness—God will come and attend us.

The Scriptures also tell us that when Jesus heard that Herod had killed his cousin John, he withdrew privately to a solitary place. He just needed to get away, to reflect perhaps, and to pray. To be alone in the silences, because it is in the silences that we can hear God.

Do you remember the story of Elijah, the great and mighty prophet, who called down fire from heaven on Mount Carmel (1 Kings 18)? It's an amazing story. Queen Jezebel had brought in her gods and her priests. She had killed many of God's prophets and priests. The people of God were turning away from him and toward Baal. Elijah had had enough. Taking the bull by the horns (so to speak), he delivered the ultimatum to the people on Mount Carmel: "You call on the name of your god, and I will call on the name of the Lord. The god who answers by fire—he is God" (18:24).

Of course, God was victorious. But then Jezebel heard about what happened and declared that she would kill Elijah. Frightened (and no doubt exhausted from this showdown), Elijah fled toward Horeb. But when he came to Beersheba, he separated himself from his servant and went a day's journey into the desert. Worn out, he sat under a tree and asked God to take his life. "I have had enough, Lord," he said. "Take my life" (19:4).

In the next verse we read these words: "Then he lay down under the tree and fell asleep."

God sent an angel to attend to Elijah, feeding him. After Elijah ate, he fell asleep again. The angel returned, this time, saying, "Get up and eat, *for the journey is too much for you*" (19:7, emphasis mine). Touched by God in such an incredible way, Elijah was able to travel for forty days and forty nights until he reached Horeb, where Mount Sinai (the mountain of God, the place where Moses received the Ten Commandments) is located. There, the Lord told Elijah to go stand on the mountain, because his presence was about to pass by.

A great and powerful wind came, but God was not in the wind.

An earthquake shook the ground, but God was not in the earthquake.

Then came a fire, but God was not in the fire.

But then . . . Elijah heard a gentle whisper. And God was in the whisper.

Shhhhh. God is speaking. Can you hear him? You can't if you are talking, or running around, or dragging yourself from the bed and then working till way past late. My good friend Robert Benson once said to me, "The only person who hears what God is whispering to your heart is *you*. But, you won't hear him if you don't hush."

"Be still," the Sons of Korah wrote in Psalm 46. "Be still and know that I am God." In another Old Testament song, we read Solomon's words, "You are a garden locked up, my sister, my bride; you are a spring enclosed, a sealed fountain" (Song of Songs 4:12).

In this part of Solomon's love poem, the bride and groom have married and have now "gone away" together. The honeymoon, so to speak. Sealed away, her plants become an orchard of pomegranates with choice fruits, with henna, nard, saffron, calamus, cinnamon, every kind of incense tree, myrrh and aloes, and all the finest spices. Take a moment to count those choice fruits. There are nine. Nine fruits budding from this time alone, enclosed and sealed.

Galatians 5:22 speaks of the fruit of the Spirit: love, joy, peace, patience, kindness, goodness, faithfulness, gentleness, and self-control. Count them; there are nine. "Those

Deb Kinnard, a reimbursement specialist from Elk Grove, Illinois, says, "I wish I didn't, but I do take naps. I nap because as I get older, it feels as though I have no choice. I get home from work about three, and by then I'm wiped out. My job is plenty stressful though it's part-time, and I attribute the tiredness partly to that. I take between thirty minutes and an hour and wake up refreshed to start supper and get on with it. I don't do anything special like put cream on my face or anything like that. I just darken the room, get horizontal, and am out in seconds."

MORE BEDDING TIPS

When it comes to your bedding, make sure you pick linens you can sleep with. If you're just not the sateen kind of gal, don't buy them, no matter how pretty you think they look on a bed. Take the time to head over to a department store and talk with an informative clerk. Check out everything from Egyptian cotton to modal to polyester to frette. If you don't have a department store nearby, go online and type "fine linens" into a search engine.

Also, when you are purchasing your bedding, be sure to look for the colors you like, but above all, note the size of your mattress. Nothing is more frustrating than trying to sleep on a sheet that doesn't fit the mattress!

who belong to Christ Jesus exhibit the fruit," Paul goes on to say. *Those who belong.*

Those who spend time with him. Restful time. Time when we lay down and allow him to nurture us and nourish us.

Refreshed, we can arise and walk on in our journey.

Questions for Personal Reflection or Group Study

1. Do you schedule time each day for a nap, however brief? If so, how have you managed it? If not, why not?
2. How important are getaways to you?
3. What is your favorite personal getaway?
4. Do you schedule quiet time with God? How important is silence in your prayer life?
5. Share a time, if you will, when God spoke to your heart out of the silence.

Here's a Valuable Tip

Aromatherapy will bring you to the "heights of relaxation." Lotions, body and linen sprays, bath oils and shower gels, potpourri oils, candles, etc., are easy to find on the shelves of drugstores, specialty stores, or online.

Key ingredients to look for are:

Lavender (can also be found in baby lotions and wipes)
Geranium
Rose
Chamomile
Clary sage
Thyme
Sandalwood
Juniper berry
Tlang ylang
Sweet marjoram

4

SPAS AND SALONS

My lover is to me a cluster of henna blossoms from the vineyards of En Gedi.

Song of Songs 1:14

In days gone by in Any Small Town, America, you would most likely find only one beauty parlor and one barbershop, the latter's exterior typically adorned with a red, white, and blue barber's pole. Nail salons, massage therapy salons, and day spas were nearly unheard of, especially to the average citizen. The rich and the famous could flit away for a few days or a week, but not Mr. and Mrs. Joe American.

Today, almost anyone can be found sitting in the hot tub of a day spa or reading a book while getting her toes trimmed and painted. Gone forever, it seems, are the "every two weeks whether you need it or not" hair trims. Today's men, women, and even teenagers are flocking to the pampering places.

Even more interesting are the locations where these places are popping up. Recently, as I trudged once again through an airport, laden with an armload of carry-on luggage, a weighty purse, and enough strain in my shoulders to make a grown man whimper, I noticed a "spa" to the left of the Concourse B/Concourse C security checkpoint. I stopped so fast I nearly toppled over. Not wanting to cause a scene jumping up and down and shouting "Glory, Hallelujah!" I moseyed on over, pulling my luggage cart behind me. As soon as I slipped out of the hustle and bustle of the main hallway and into the glassed-in structure of the salon, instrumental music filled my senses. The stresses of life were momentarily halted while I scanned the "pleasure buffet" and price list. It included everything from massages (which I needed) to manicures (which I didn't need) to pedicures (which I needed) and finally, cosmetics. This was a miniature full-service type of spa.

"May I help you?" a pretty young clerk inquired.

I told her that, yes, I thought she just might be able to help me. "I've been in a lot of pain across my shoulders for several weeks," I told her.

"And pulling luggage doesn't help," she sympathized.

"No, it doesn't." Ah, the joy of finding an understanding soul.

"Would you like a fifteen-minute or thirty-minute chair massage?" she asked.

I glanced at my watch. I had plenty of time, but I opted for the fifteen minute. She instructed me to "sign here and have a seat," which I happily did. I was nearly as giddy as a child on Christmas Eve waiting to hear the sound of reindeer on the rooftop. Only, in my case, I anxiously awaited the sound of my own name.

"Eva?" another attractive clerk said, approaching me. She gave my hand a firm shake as she introduced herself. I thought, *Good handshake. Strong hands.* The possibility of a massage to die for was looking way up.

Jan Davis Warren, a homemaker from Owasso, Oklahoma, says, "I go every other week for a facial—because I'm over fifty and I like the Christian woman who does the service, and I got a great package price. It all started when my daughter and I went to a women's show in Tulsa they have once a year at the Expo. We met this woman who had a booth and was offering a special for microderm. I purchased two sets of three sessions of microdermabrasions. One for me and one for my daughter. Even had my eyelashes curled with a permanent solution like you use to curl your hair. Lasted for about six weeks, and since she tinted the lashes too I didn't have to put on mascara or curl my lashes for almost that long. She uses all top-of-the-market products from Calamari masks to biogenie treatments."

Fifteen minutes later, I was a changed woman. The price wasn't bad either, especially considering where I was. As I said my good-byes to the staff and headed toward security, I whistled a little tune, happy to be alive . . . and pain free.

The Body Beautiful—Physical

> You are a garden fountain, a well of flowing water streaming down from Lebanon.
>
> Song of Songs 4:15

What can make us feel more pampered than the time we spend getting a pedicure, a manicure, our hair trimmed and styled, or any of the vast number of indulgences found within the walls of a spa?

Did you know that the Dead Sea, located in the southernmost part of Israel, has a higher content of salt and minerals than any other body of water in the world?

People come from all around the world just to bathe and float in its slick waters, rub its mineral-rich mud on their skin, or indulge in a stay in any of the fine hotel/spas along its shoreline.

Some of the most famous people in history, including Cleopatra, have known of its curative powers.

www.deadsea.co.il/ENA/Index.html

But, with so many out there, how's a girl to know which one to pick? What are the different types of salons and spas one can enter . . . for a day, a weekend, or even an extended period of time?

Spas

Do you know where the term *spa* began?

The word *spa* derives from a Belgian town whose springs supposedly had the power to cure. So, originally, when you thought "spa," you would have thought "water." For people like me who love the feel of a shower's spray over their face or the quiet moments immersed in water (whether in a bath or swimming pool), the "healing qualities" of water come as no surprise.

There are different kinds of "waters" in which to find those cures we are in search of. Mineral springs contain . . . well, minerals, along with various salts. Thermal, or hot, springs also contain minerals, but it's the heat from the water that induces relaxation, relieves pain, and improves circulation.

One of the things that draws us to spas is the franticness of our daily lives versus the calm and serenity found within these temporary moments of paradise.

The types of services you might find are:

Massage (full body, back, foot, head, etc.)
Skin care
Body wraps
Thermal hot baths
Cold baths
Saunas
Reflecting pools
Acupuncture
Manicures and pedicures
Exercise facilities and fitness classes
Hair care

Prices, of course, vary from less than a hundred dollars to so much more than that.

Salons

Salons today have as much to do with the whole body experience as they do with hair. It is rare indeed to find "just" a hair salon. Yesterday as I searched for a nail salon, I came across a sparkling new one just two miles from my home. Inside I was faced with a choice of having a manicure, pedicure, facial, waxing, mircrodermabrasion, massage, or permanent makeup tattooed on. (I can't even begin to imagine doing the latter.)

Short on time, I elected to have just a pedicure. I was quickly taken to a private room (with a mounted television and wine rack with crystal stemware, no less, where I could be served one—but no more than one—cocktail after 5:00 p.m.) and placed in a chair designed to massage the back of my body (can you say "ahhhh," boys and girls?) while my feet soaked in a whirlpool. I was treated to a "foot mash" and lower-leg treatment as well. (By the way, I passed on the cocktail.)

This was a far cry from a recent experience while I was traveling through a small town. Wanting to purchase some hair product, I looked in the yellow pages of the phone book, then drove down a little side street until I spied the handmade sign hanging from just beyond the door, indicating that I'd found the right place. I parked my rental car and, seconds later, entered the door that was more window than wood. I couldn't help but smile when I gained my focus from the strong sunlight outside to the fluorescent bulbs inside. A line of about four salon chairs faced a long wall of mirrors, which were mostly adorned with photographs and certificates.

Nothing, but nothing, screamed "posh salon." There was no decorative shelving stocked with product, no ornately framed prints, no statues or floral arrangements. And yet I understand this particular hair salon is one of the busiest in the area. If you need an appointment for the near future, you're probably out of luck! You'll only get your hair done here, so if you need anything more, anything "extra," you'd best keep looking.

Most salons today are appealing because of their ability to do more than hair. They boast of tanning beds, pedicures, manicures, massages, body scrubs, facials, cosmetic centers . . . well, the works. Some have a few services and some have a lot. You'll find walls painted in soothing colors and decorated with paintings and other fashionable artwork, furniture to die for, and personnel who are well trained to make you feel like the most special person in the world.

Costly (or more costly than your "just give me a hair-cut" salon) is not always better. While it's true that the more pricey salons employ only the best hairstylists, etc., it doesn't mean you can't find a really good stylist, cosmetician, or nail tech at one less frou-frou.

In spite of my husband's claim that I'm high maintenance, the salon I visit about every six weeks is small but comfortable, nicely decorated but not posh, and very reasonably priced. The owner, a lovely woman named Marissa, is not only the proprietor, she is *the* hairstylist. For a very reasonable price you can get cut, curled, permed, colored, highlighted, styled, blown dry, and even waxed. (Your body, not your hair!) She is very good at her job and booked so far in advance that I shudder when I realize I failed to make an appointment after my last trim.

When it comes to spas and salons, author and speaker Pam Farrel, author of *Red Hot Monogamy*, says, "You can create a spa-like atmosphere at home. Splurge on a massage showerhead and plenty of plush white towels and matching white robes with his and her monograms. For pennies you can buy soothing instrumental music. Place a cooler of lemon water in the refrigerator. Buy a wide variety of lotions, bath salts, and scrubs. I also enjoy the spa at home day alone as well. A mask, face peel, pedicure, manicure, a long bath, an afternoon of reading on the chaise lounge on the patio with some chilled herb tea or lemon water with some soothing harp music playing in the background is great medicine to lessen the effects of a stressful week. However, nothing is as restoring as gathering my favorite devotionals, my well-worn Bible, and favorite praise CDs and cozying up in my robe for a leisurely morning away with God. Keeping in touch with my Creator reignites and rejuvenates my heart."

Frou-frou doesn't always mean better. Take a group of women—any group of women—sit them at a table, and ask them if they've had a bad salon experience, and listen to the stories fly! You'll also find that many of the stories come from the more expensive salons.

Which brings me to my next point: finding the right salon for you. And, it is imperative that you do. (Some women swear that finding a new salon is right up there with finding a new gynecologist. It's enough to make a grown woman cry!) Just because your grandmother or your best friend swears by a particular salon or stylist does not mean you'll be happy with their choice. In the end, it's all about trial and error. When you do find the salon created, it seems, just for you, stay with it as long as you can.

The Body Beautiful—Spiritual

Come, all you who are thirsty, come to the waters . . . and without cost.

Isaiah 55:1

Life is hard, make no mistake about it. And it seems that it keeps getting harder all the time.

It's not just our physical bodies that take the beating but our spiritual bodies as well. We look for little ways—and even big ways—to renew and revive ourselves. Ways that, in the midst of hardship, will draw us closer to almighty God.

The lowest place on the earth's surface is the Dead Sea, a body of water located in the southern part of Israel and filled with twelve billion tons of salt. If our tears of sorrow were to be counted within its waters, it would account for an awful lot of heartache.

Yet, on either side of this lowest point are mountain ranges—high points—including one of the most beautiful oases in the world.

One of those "points" is a place known as En Gedi, which is, in reality, no more than a severely gorged mountain range. Located six hundred feet above the Dead Sea, it acts as an aqueduct, bringing a wealth of water to the region. Pleasant year-round climate and the abundant springs provide fertile conditions for lush agriculture such as tall date palms and tropical (Sudanian) plants and Mediterranean and Steppian flora such as the exquisite willow.

> ## OASIS
>
> 1. a fertile or green area in an arid region (as a desert)
> 2. something that provides refuge, relief, or pleasant contrast
>
> Ref: Merriam Webster Online

It was to En Gedi that the young shepherd who would be king, David, took refuge when running from King Saul, a madman . . . *and* his father-in-law. Because of his popularity among the peoples from even the surrounding nations, David was able to slip from one area to the next, gaining a band of followers as he went.

It must have been difficult, having done nothing wrong and yet living on the run. No place to call home, the wife of his youth left behind in the palace (and eventually married to someone else), a bunch of ragtag folks under his responsibility, and a madman hot on his trail.

In 1 Samuel 23 we read, "David went up from there and lived in the strongholds of En Gedi."

One look at photos taken in En Gedi will help explain why David was able to feel as though he could take refuge there, to feel protected by God, and to regain his momentum. If nothing else, he could have stood beneath any of the number of waterfalls bursting from the hillsides, perhaps even the one carrying his name today, Nahal David.

Later, when Saul followed David to En Gedi, the king went into one of the numerous caves dotting the mountainside for the purpose of "relieving himself." Unbeknownst to him, David was in the cave. While Saul was doing whatever he needed to do, David took out a knife and cut a piece of the king's robe. Close enough to kill the man who wrongly pursued him and yet in touch enough with God not to.

> Whoever believes in me, as the Scripture has said, streams of living water will flow from within him.
>
> John 7:38

When Saul and his army were leaving the immediate area, David stepped out of the cave and called down to Saul, showing him the evidence of his love and devotion. After this display, and for a while, Saul left David alone.

A thousand or so years later, the Son of David (Jesus) referred to himself as "living water."

One of the most endearing stories for women is Christ's encounter with the woman at the well (John 4). This unknown woman (and she could be *any* of us) had come to the well in the heat of the day. In fact, John stresses this point. Most women went for water in the cool of the day, whether the early morning hours or in the evening. But this woman, we later learn, might have been socially outcast because of the number of marriages she'd had and the fact that she was now living with a man who was not her legal spouse. For this reason, she may have chosen to come in the heat of the day rather than in the cool of the day, preferring the scorch of the sun to the snide remarks and sideward glances.

And so Jesus met her "where she was." Since it was the noon hour and he'd walked all the way from Judea, he was no doubt hot and thirsty, and—the Bible tells us—tired. Physically, he needed water. He sent his disciples into town to buy food while he sat at the well known as Jacob's Well. The Samaritan woman approached, no doubt carrying her water pitchers. One can only imagine the thoughts that ran through her mind as she saw Jesus sitting there. Perhaps she stalled for a moment, slowing her steps. Perhaps she took a deep breath, pressed her lips together in anticipation, but then—knowing what must be done—continued forward. Perhaps she thought, *If I ignore him, maybe he won't bother me* or *If I close my eyes, maybe he won't see me.*

"Will you give me a drink?" Jesus asked her.

The woman was stunned. Not only was this man a Jew (Jews and Samaritans weren't known for socializing together), but he was also a teacher, or rabbi. Men didn't teach women, nor would they typically speak to them in public places.

> Jesus answered her, "If you knew the gift of God and who it is that asks you for a drink, you would have asked him and he would have given you living water."
>
> "Sir," the woman said, "you have nothing to draw with and the well is deep. Where can you get this living water? Are you greater than our father Jacob, who gave us the well and drank from it himself, as did also his sons and his flocks and herds?"
>
> Jesus answered, "Everyone who drinks this water will be thirsty again, but whoever drinks the water I give him will never thirst. Indeed, the water I give him will become in him a spring of water welling up to eternal life."
>
> John 4:10–14

Jesus of the New Testament has so often been compared to Moses of the Old Testament. And well he should be. Jesus came to finish the work of his servant Moses. As the people under Rome's thumb in Christ's day were spiritually thirsty, those Moses had led out of Egyptian captivity were physically thirsty.

In Exodus 17 we read the story of the wandering Hebrews—already filled with manna from heaven—as they left the Desert of Sin to camp at a place known as Rephidim. Once there, they realized there was no water, and, naturally, they began to whine and complain. "Give us water to drink," they demanded of Moses, as though he could ride his camel down to the nearest convenience store and purchase a few hundred thousand gallons.

> For I will pour water on the thirsty land, and streams on the dry ground; I will pour out my Spirit on your offspring, and my blessing on your descendants.
>
> Isaiah 44:3

When Moses warned them that they were putting the Lord to the test, they continued their complaining, asking, "Why did you bring us up out of Egypt to make us and our children and livestock die of thirst?"

Moses took the situation to the Lord, and God answered him. "Walk on ahead of the people. Take with you some of the elders of Israel and take in your hand the staff with which you struck the Nile, and go. I will stand there before you by the rock at Horeb. [Author's note: also known as "The Mountain of God."] Strike the rock, and water will come out of it for the people to drink" (Exod. 17:5–6).

And, of course, this is exactly what happened.

We all need places such as En Gedi, or Horeb, or Jacob's Well, but they don't have to be long distances away, and, as Isaiah wrote in 55:1, they don't have to be costly. We need a place where we can go to find rest. A place where God can meet us, wash us, refresh us.

When David was in the Desert of Judah, he wrote: "God, you are my God, earnestly I seek you; my soul thirsts for you, my body longs for you, in a dry and weary land where there is no water" (Ps. 63:1).

In Hebrew, David's word for *earnestly* is *shachar*, which means "to seek early" or "early in the morning." Reading this, we can get a sense that—before the rest of his world woke up and began making demands upon him—David went to those quiet places within and without and meditated on God. As a poet, perhaps he did what we today call "journaling," penning poems and songs of love and devotion. These may well have been the times, as the sun began its daily climb over the rocky crags around him, that David paused to draw from the well that would never, ever run dry.

The desire to be with God, to know him, and to draw from him is among our most primal. Yet, we do more than desire him. We *need* him. Just as we cannot live without water, we cannot live without God's presence. For those who seek him, it is a spiritually insatiable need. We fill up and are dipped into the cool liquid and must return to the water again and again. The more dry and weary we are, the more we need to return.

> As the deer pants for streams of water, so my soul pants for you, O God. My soul thirsts for God, for the living God. When can I go and meet with God?
>
> Psalm 42:1–2

When Moses went to the Mountain of God, he was told to take with him the staff already in his hand and, with that staff, to "strike the rock." God also told him that he would *meet* Moses at the rock. Just as, years later, he *met* the woman at the well.

63

Ane Mulligan, a drama director and freelance writer from Suwanee, Georgia, says, "If you are going to a spa or salon for hair removal, allow me to tell you my story. A few years ago I decided I was sick and tired of shaving my legs, so I bought an Epilady. You know, that torture thing some *man* thought up? But it worked. I used it for about three years, until I noticed I didn't have any more hair on my legs. WAHOO!"

Perhaps it is no mistake that Jesus is so often called the rock of our salvation. So willing to meet us where we are and to fill us, surround us even, with water.

Living water. And so free. So very, very free. Nothing frou-frou. No appointments necessary. Just a willing heart and a thirsty soul.

Questions for Personal Reflection or Group Study

1. Have you ever been to a spa/salon, whether for a few hours, a day, or several days?
2. What "drove" you to go?
3. Does water draw you, whether in the form of the ocean, a pool, a bath, or a spa?
4. Reread Isaiah 55:1 and John 4:10. Note the words *without money and without cost* (Isaiah) and *gift* (John). In the financially difficult times of the biblical days, even water had to be purchased. Knowing this, what do you think Isaiah and Jesus were trying to say about the "free" gift of "water"?[1]
5. Read Revelation 21:6 and 22:17. What do these verses say to you?

Here's a Valuable Tip

Be cautious in your choice of salon; they are popping up all over the place, so you have many options. Before you trust anyone with your body, make sure the establishment has a current business license. Be savvy enough to ask questions about the products they use for cleaning their instruments. The salon experience should be about getting pampered, not about getting an infection.

Though they often are the brunt of jokes, low-price hair salons (typically found as franchises) are not always bad. As I stated before, you can have a bad experience anywhere, whether the simple trim runs you five dollars or fifty. If your money is tight, look in the yellow pages for one of the following franchise hair salons.[2]

Fantastic Sams
Great Clips
Hair Cuttery
Supercuts
The Lemon Tree

When it comes to lower-priced salons that do the full-body treatment, again, they're popping up everywhere. Do your homework. Ask for a tour. Study their price sheet carefully. Call the Better Business Bureau before you make any decisions. By all means, if you have a bad feeling about the place, go with your instincts.

5

MASSAGE

Jesus reached out his hand and touched the man. "I am willing," he said. "Be clean!" Immediately he was cured.

Matthew 8:3

My first experience with massage began with the Super Bowl. My husband and I had been invited to the home of some friends for the annual party. We arrived and did what the other couples did—separated. Guys in front of the big screen, gals around the kitchen table, sipping on hot coffee and nibbling on all the goodies. At some point, I got up and felt the small of my back "give way." I limped a bit to the living room for the halftime show, and by the time I arrived I felt like my old self. A few minutes later—entertained for another year—I headed back to the kitchen with the other wives, where we ate more food and drank more coffee. And, of course, gabbed.

When the game was over, the men joined us women. My husband finally asked, "You ready to go?" and I said, "Yes." Thanking the host and hostess, I got up and again felt my back give way. Somehow I made it to our car, but the ride home was agony. By the time I got to our bed, I was ready to cry. Three days later, I was still miserable. A friend called her massage therapist, who happened to live in my neighborhood. He arrived and opened up his little portable table, but my pain was to the point where I couldn't even sit up much less walk to it. Like the hero he's always been, my husband lifted me in his arms and carried me to it. As I positioned my face into the "face hole," I felt the pain of my lower back release a bit. An hour later, I could walk to the sofa, though not much farther. A couple of days later, the visit was repeated until, after about a week, I was an upright human again.

That day I learned firsthand about the healing power of touch; I've been a loyal "customer" ever since.

The Body Beautiful—Physical

> He touched her hand and the fever left her, and she got up and began to wait on him.
>
> Matthew 8:15

Kathryn Porter, a stay-at-home mom from Colorado Springs and author of *Too Much Stuff: Decluttering Your Heart and Home*, says, "Massages can crimp a tight budget; massage therapy schools offer alternatives to women who lack the extra funds for this treat. Massages run twenty-five dollars instead of fifty. The main difference is the environment. The school is not as aesthetically pleasing as the room of most licensed masseuses, but the massage is still good."

Massage therapists (sometimes known as masseuses or masseurs) carry what is known as a "license to touch." Don't you just love the sound of that? Allow me to say it again: *license to touch.* In many states this means that the Department of Health/Department of Quality Assurance has licensed professionals such as massage therapists, chiropractors, osteopathologists, doctors, nurses, and physical therapists to heal through their power of touch.

When it comes to massage (or massage therapy, as I like to call it), there are literally hundreds of modalities in which a professional can specialize. However, the four most commonly sought after are:

1. Swedish

The most requested and performed massage is known simply as "Swedish." A Swedish doctor named Per Henrik Ling developed Swedish massage in the 1700s. (Yeah, that long ago.) Its main purpose is to increase the blood's oxygen flow while at the same time releasing toxins held by muscles. Additionally, Swedish massage stimulates the skin and nervous system, soothes the nerves, reduces stress, and is suggested in a regular program for stress management.[1]

2. Deep Tissue

Deep tissue massage works more with the neuromuscular/skeletal junctures. In other words, it goes down to where the muscle attaches to the bones. In doing so, it releases the chronic patterns of tension. Therapists who perform deep tissue massage use slow strokes and deep finger pressure. Sometimes the therapy may actually cause the patient some pain either during or after treatment; however, it doesn't last long.

3. Neuromuscular

Also known as "trigger point therapy," neuromuscular massage involves applying pressure to the knots (or "trigger points") in order to relieve the pain. The interesting thing about trigger points is that while they may be located in a specific part of the body, the pain actually occurs elsewhere. Therefore, if the trigger point (or knot) is pressed, the pain is felt in another part of the body rather than within the "knotted" muscle.

Trigger Point Therapy is not new; Dr. Janet Travell developed it more than sixty years ago.

4. Hot Stone/Hot Rocks

Hot stone therapy is the newest fad, for lack of a better word. In this "hands off" therapy, various sizes of basalt (volcanic) stones or rocks (which retain heat well) are heated and then applied to specific points on the body. This action, in turn, melts away painful knots as it dissolves tension and stress. Hot stone therapy is also used as a massage tool.

Removing the Stigma

For many years, "massage" was associated with "parlors," or places where men would go for reasons we won't talk about here. Typically, today's massage therapists are trained and licensed. They operate their businesses under strict rules established by health codes. (Again, this is not to say that *all* have a license. Some states do not require a license. Anyone who thinks he or she can give a "good rub" can hang out a shingle and frame their first earned dollar. You should know your state's requirements and ask to see a diploma from a reputable school and a business license. This is truly *your* responsibility.)

You should also be wise enough to know that male massage therapists are *not* "all gay." (In fact, the two massage therapists I've used on a consistent basis are a man and woman who are married to each other and are parents and grandparents-to-be!) This is as ridiculous as saying that all male hairdressers are gay. It's labeling and it's wrong, and you'll do yourself a great disservice if you believe it to be true.

There's another stigma that goes along with massage therapy, and that is that massage therapy is a part of the New Age culture. While it's true that many massage therapists will talk to you about the benefits of holistic medicine, it is not true that they are sucking you into some type of cultic religion. (My gynecologist is Jewish and my cardiologist is Hindu, but that doesn't mean I'll be leaving my Christian beliefs behind on account of them.)

In reality, massage therapy is very much in tune to the divine nature of God because it's about touch and energy. Allow me to explain it to you the way my massage therapist explained it to me as we nibbled on Italian food at a little eatery one rainy afternoon. She said:

> ## THE BENEFITS OF MASSAGE
>
> - Increased blood flow brings nutrients and oxygen to the body.
> - Strengthens the immune system.
> - Relaxes the muscles and relieves stress.
> - In cases of inactivity, massage therapy exercises the muscles.
> - Brings relief to painful joints.
> - Brings faster healing to injured muscles and/or joints.
> - Reduces depression.
> - Reduces blood pressure.
>
> Reference: www.holistic-online.com/massage/mas_benefits.htm

Have you ever entered a room in which two people had been arguing? You can just feel it in the air, can't you? That's because we—as human beings—are made up of energy. It's that energy that gives us our vitality, or life. That energy can be traced down to the electrical impulses within us that are constant and steady. [Think: heartbeat and nerve endings.] When they cease to be constant and steady, our physical bodies have died.

That energy responds to the elements of God's good gifts on earth, using our senses to do so. Sight, hearing, smell, taste, and . . . *touch*. This is how our heavenly Father created us. We see something beautiful and are enraptured. We hear a symphony and are enthralled. We smell a deliciously home-cooked meal and are suddenly hungry. Or, the scent of lavender can make us sleepy. When we taste a yummy dessert (and I'm just speaking from personal experience here), we feel content inside (not to mention a few pounds heavier).

And then we have touch. A slap across the face comes across quite differently than a stroke on the cheek, doesn't it? Touch, for humans, is essential. We can live without sight or hearing. We can make do without smell or taste. But think about life *without* touch. It's one of the very first things a baby responds to, and our need for it continues until the day we die.

A touch "done right" can heal, both physically and emotionally. When I was charge nurse in a nursing home, one of the things I chose to do was go into each patient's room at least once during my shift and to touch them. To rub their backs. To stroke their arms. To caress their faces or to hold their hands. So many of them had been abandoned by their family members. For me, the idea that they would die in that place never having another human being lovingly touch them was unthinkable. And so I touched. They, in turn, responded.

Positively.

When it comes to massage, author and speaker Kathleen Jackson (*The Godly Business Woman Magazine Guide to Cooking and Entertainment*) says, "Massages force me to shut down for an hour or so. I always seem to spend this time talking to God. My favorite type of massage is hot rock massage, a deep, penetrating massage that really gets down and works out the little knots."

The Body Beautiful—Spiritual

And wherever he went—into villages, towns or country-side—they placed the sick in the marketplaces. They begged him to let them touch even the edge of his cloak, and all who touched him were healed.

Mark 6:56

To touch God.

To be touched *by* God.

What could be better than this?

When Jesus ministered during his time on earth, people came from all over to touch him and to be touched by him in order that they might be healed. Mothers and fathers brought their young children just for the privilege of having their Creator's touch upon them once again.

Jesus healed through the power of his Holy Spirit and by touching those who were afflicted by both physical disease and sin.

The Gospels of Matthew, Mark, and Luke tell the story of the temple ruler named Jairus who came to Jesus, asking that the Healer come to his home for the purpose of *touching* his dead daughter. Mark's writing records it like this: "My little daughter is dying. Please come and put your hands on her so that she will be healed and live" (5:23).

All he wanted from Jesus was a touch—"put your hands on her."

Naturally, Jesus got up and left with the ruler, followed by the disciples and a large crowd of people who, I'm sure, were anxious to see what this new and unorthodox teacher would be doing next.

Before he could get very far, a woman who had been bleeding for twelve years managed to get close enough to Jesus. She believed that if she could just *touch* his clothes (just his clothes!), she would be healed.

It's important to know that, due to the culture of the Jewish people during this era, this woman—because of her bleeding—would have been considered ceremonially unclean and therefore untouchable. This woman hadn't been allowed to touch or be touched in twelve long, agonizing years.

When the woman was able to brush her fingers along the hem of his garment, Jesus stopped. He'd felt a power go out of him, so much so that he asked, "Who touched me?"

The disciples must have chuckled a bit at their leader's question. "There are people crowding all around you! Of course someone has touched you" (paraphrase, mine).

But Jesus kept looking around until the woman came to him, knelt down, and told him what she had done. Instead of rebuking her, he called her his own. "Daughter," he said, "your faith has healed you. Go in peace" (Mark 5:34).

Jesus then went on to the home of Jairus, where—in the interim—the little girl had died. "Don't bother the Teacher," they told her father. "Your little girl is dead."

Jesus turned to the ruler and said, "Don't be afraid. Just believe." He went into the home, took the girl by the hand, and said, "*Talitha koum!*" (*Talitha koum* is Aramaic, the common language of Jesus' day. It means, "Little girl, I say to you, get up!")

At his touch, and upon hearing his words, the little girl got up.

One of the witnesses to this miracle was the disciple named John. Years later, John would write these words in his first letter to the believers. "That which was from the beginning, which we have heard, which we have seen with our eyes, which we have looked at and our hands have *touched*—this we proclaim concerning the Word of life" (1 John 1:1, emphasis mine).

John is not talking about being touched *by* Jesus but rather having *touched* him.

When I think about that verse of Scripture, two key moments come to mind. The first took place just before the betrayal and crucifixion of the Messiah. The Twelve were in the upper room with Jesus having the Passover seder meal. Jesus told those around the table that one of them would betray him before the night was over. Of course the men who had loved him and followed him unconditionally for more than three years were quite perplexed and maybe even a bit horrified. They looked from one to the other. Then, John—who was reclining next to Jesus (in those days people reclined on their elbows toward the table rather than sitting in chairs)—leaned himself back *against* Jesus (John 13:25). "Leaned against" the text says. So close that, perhaps, he could feel or hear the Savior's heartbeat. But most definitely, his head was against Jesus' chest. Touching him as if the mindful part of John was now privy to the heartbeat of the Creator.

The second moment came after the resurrection of the Christ. The disciples were together in a room, tucked safely behind a locked door, when suddenly Jesus was in the room, saying, "Peace be with you!"

Naturally the boys were a bit taken aback. But Jesus said, "Why are you troubled and why do doubts rise in your minds? Look at my hands and my feet. It is I myself! *Touch* me and see" (Luke 24:39, emphasis mine).

Touch me.

Oh, to have been John in that moment . . . in either of those moments! To have touched . . . *Jesus!* And to have been touched in return.

When we touch Jesus or when he touches us, we are open to receiving healing and peace and—so beautifully—being called his daughter. When we take a moment to touch him by leaning our heads against his chest, we just might be privy to hearing his heartbeat.

What could be more healing than that?

Questions for Personal Reflection or Group Study

1. Do you get massages? Why or why not?
2. If you do get massages, what is your favorite type? Why?
3. How important is touching, whether as the giver or the receiver?
4. What does it mean to you to be "touched by God"?
5. What does it mean to you to "touch God"?

Rose McCauley, a retired elementary school teacher from Cynthiana, Kentucky, says, "I get massages, usually one a month. They help my muscle pain and also help open up my sinuses when the therapist uses the hot stones."

Here's a Valuable Tip

I cannot stress this point enough: before you enter a massage salon or spa for the first time, ask to see the business license. Ask questions that will ensure that the person doing the massage is both qualified and educated.

6

SKIN PROTECTION

Do not stare at me because I am dark, because I am darkened by the sun.

Song of Songs 1:6

Something stirs inside whenever I hear Celtic music. It is always oddly familiar, even if I have never heard that particular piece before, as though it is able to resonate within my ancestry.

One look at me and it isn't difficult to figure out why. My ancestry is Irish. I have red highlights in my hair (even when I'm not applying it from a bottle), a fair complexion, and freckles on nearly every inch of my body. Time outdoors means lots of sunscreen, both to protect my lily white and to keep the possibility of cancer at bay.

When it comes to my skin, I was born caught between the proverbial rock and hard place. In the Deep South (where I learned how to properly fry a chicken and swoon at all the appropriate times), ladies of means were often noted by the fairness of their skin. A true lady of the South wouldn't be caught dead working or sweating in direct sunlight.

(My aunt always said, "Ladies in the South don't sweat, darlin', they glow.") In days gone by, even a walk along the avenue with her favorite beau required a parasol (preferably one that matched her dress) arched perfectly over her head. Those ladies who enjoyed gardening—or perhaps fishing—did so in the cool of the morning or evening and even then wore wide-brimmed straw hats, sometimes with funny flowers or birds perched about.

But I was also a child born along the Georgia coastline in the 1950s. This meant spending a great deal of time during my childhood on the beaches or the thick banks of the numerous lakes and creeks where blankets were spread and laughter drifted through the rushes of the marsh and the giant oaks. These were the days of the Coppertone ad. You remember it, don't you? A cute little puppy pulls at the back of a little girl's frilly underpants, exposing the stark white of her derriere against the rich tan of her back. These were also the days of such idiotic measures as combining Mercurochrome (or iodine) and baby oil in order to achieve the perfect tan.

Being of Irish descent, of course, I would burn to a toasty crisp if I wasn't extremely careful and attentive to my skin's needs. I vividly recall the older women who lived on the beaches where we spent so many of my growing-up days. Their skin had taken on a leathery appearance, like that of an old farm animal . . . or a lizard, even. When I asked my mother about it, she replied, "They've spent too much time in the sun." Even as a child I knew this wasn't attractive and that I didn't want to look like this . . . ever. Even if it meant forfeiting the desired California Tan look.

As I got older and began traveling to our nation's chillier landscapes in winter months, I learned that the cold is just as harsh on the skin's appearance. Protecting the skin, however, goes much deeper than merely attempting to look

> Kim Sawyer, a teacher and author from Hutchinson, Kansas, says, "My favorite skin protection is Oil of Olay lotion with SPF 15—moisturizes and protects at the same time. Part of the reason I started wearing SPF every day was to protect myself from the ultraviolet lighting in stores—it was hard on my lupus. I have been healed of lupus, but the moisturizer is still great for the skin."

good. We now know how unhealthy too much of nature's heat and cold can be to the overall health of our bodies.

The Body Beautiful—Physical

I have seen all the things that are done under the sun; all of them are meaningless, a chasing after the wind.

Ecclesiastes 1:14

When I was a child it was as simple as my asking, "Why does her skin look like that?" and Mother answering, "Too much time in the sun."

Could it *get* any less complex?

Today, however, we're talking about solar radiation, free radical damage, and UV rays. We read about the ozone layer . . . and are concerned! Not so much with the condition of the world, though surely that's important. Oh no. Our vain little selves are more worried about what it means to *us*. Especially those us-es who are over thirty.

Tanning

Okay, so let's be honest. What looks better than a little color on the skin, especially for those of us who are not "by

God, of color"? When I do manage to spend some time in the glorious sunlight (such as those precious hours spent in the swimming pool with my granddaughter)—enough to garner what (if you saw my torso, you'd know) could be called a tan—I often hear from family and friends, "You look healthy."

In the 1920s, French designer Coco Chanel decreed the tan to be a fashionably acceptable look.

It can all be so confusing! To tan or not to tan, *that* is the question. Does one lie out or does one lie "in" (as in a tanning bed)? Or, does one avoid the sun at all costs? (Providing, of course, you have not already suffered from any form of skin cancer or been told by your doctor to stay clear of that glowing round thing in the sky.)

First, let's understand the different types of sun rays.

There are three different types of UV rays: UVC, UVA, and UVB. UVC rays are the most damaging, so we're going to look at them first. Fortunately, the ozone layer protects us from UVC rays, keeping us from being fry babies. Unfortunately, the ozone layer has been threatened by chlorofluorocarbons (CFCs). But on the flip side, in 1987 a number of countries including the United States signed a treaty known as the Montreal Protocol, which called for the cessation of production of products containing CFCs in hopes of reducing the threat to the ozone. Scientists believe that we should be fairly "safe and sound" by 2010. (Now, don't you feel better?)

UVA rays are not blocked by the ozone layer. Out of the three, UVA is the least damaging, but that hardly keeps it from being harmless. UVA is the culprit behind premature aging (boo-hiss!). It can damage blood vessels and even affect our DNA.

UVB rays are not entirely blocked by the ozone layer, but are by 99 percent. They are more prevalent in summer and affect only the outer layer of skin. Before you breathe a sigh of relief thinking that means they're harmless, you should know that UVB rays cause sunburn faster and are the major cause of melanoma (skin cancer).

So, then, what about tanning beds? Well, if that just isn't the question of the hour. According to industry estimates, twenty-eight million Americans are tanning indoors annually at about twenty-five thousand tanning salons around the country.[1] Though the light that tanning beds yield does not come directly from the sun, they still emit UV light. It has been said—and even by myself—that once the skin has a little tan (after the superficial portion of the skin, or the epidermis, has been exposed and thereby caused the production of melanin) then the skin has a layer of protection from the sun. While this is true to some extent, it is minor protection.

In the 1970s, medical devices that emit principally UVA were developed and quickly adopted for modern indoor tanning. The biological effects of UVA were less obvious than those of UVB, which is responsible for skin reddening, or UVC, and these devices were touted as offering a "safe" tan. Today indoor tanning beds, etc., use a combination of UVA and UVB lights, simulating the mixture found in the sun.

Tanning and Cancer

Since 1894, when P. G. Unna of Berlin published a report on the connection between sunlight and cancer, volumes of studies have been released. UV radiation, whether from exposure to the sun or visits to the local tanning salon, seems to be the culprit behind the cause of the three most common skin cancers: basal cell carcinoma (BCC), squamous cell carcinoma (SCC), and melanoma. If diagnosed, a patient may actually have to remember their history of sun exposure all the way back to their childhood.

The most common form of skin cancer is BCC. Approximately 800,000 Americans are diagnosed each year with BCC. The second most common—coming in at 200,000 new cases—is SCC. Those who have a history of prolonged sun exposure, have fair skin or light hair, or have blue, green, or gray eyes are at the highest risks of contracting BCC or SCC. Finally, approximately 51,000 new cases of melanoma are reported each year to the American Medical Association. Melanoma is the most dangerous of the skin cancers and yet the most curable. If left alone, it could easily spread to other parts of the body, become difficult to treat, and then become deadly.[2]

Tanning and Wrinkles

Sometimes when we're young, the last thing we worry about is skin cancer. We don't worry about too much of anything, if we're honest about it. Skin cancer can pretty much fall into the same category as any cancer: we'll think about it and do something about it when we're older.

It's easy to feel the same way about wrinkles.

Not too long ago, I was in a restaurant where the average age of the servers and other staff seemed to be between eighteen and twenty-five. I couldn't help but notice their complexions, especially their faces. Eyes danced and teased with nary a show of crow's-feet. Lips spread in wide grins as they spoke to one another without a single wrinkle creeping up their cheekbones. I can safely estimate that nine out of ten of them were beautifully tanned.

Dropping my chin onto the ball of my fist, I declared to my dinner mate, "Look at them. Not a single sign of aging. I'd be willing to bet that not a one of them applied moisturizer this morning, nor will they before they go to bed tonight."

"Wrinkles," said my friend, "are the farthest thing from their minds."

I looked back at her and gave a wry smile. "Yeah. I remember those days. When did we get to be so old?"

Though we'll talk more about moisturizers for our faces later, be sure to note that exposure to the sun does increase wrinkles and signs of aging on our bodies. The sun's heat, though it feels good on our skin, is actually drawing out the skin's supply of natural oils. These oils keep skin young and wrinkle free.

Sun Protection Factor

SPF is the commonly used abbreviation for sun protection factor as it relates to sunscreens, which block UV rays from burning the skin at a higher rate than without sunscreen. The numbers correlate to the amount of time a person is able to stay in the sun with the sunscreen versus without it. For example, SPF 15 means a person can play or stay in the sun 15 times longer than without sunscreen.

Sunscreens—like most things in life—have practical application tips to ensure they work to their highest potential.

1. Apply about twenty minutes before you go out in the sun.
2. Remember to reapply often.
3. Don't think that just because you applied a higher SPF you don't have to reapply. Even a high SPF can

be sweated or wiped off, especially during work or play.

If you do sunburn, there's both good news and bad news. The bad news is, there's no cure. With a fair complexion and my fair share of sunburns, I can tell you that I've tried just about everything to combat the pain and swelling of a severe burn (right down to putting baking soda in a tub of water and letting the combination "pull" the sting out. It worked, but this was truly more painful than childbirth!). Cool baths, compresses, and moisturizers will also help as well as cooling gels, etc. However, if you develop a fever or chills (as I did once), upset stomach, or confusion, you must consult your physician.

> SPF relates only to UVB rays.

The Body Beautiful—Spiritual

> But let all who take refuge in you be glad; let them ever sing for joy. Spread your protection over them, that those who love your name may rejoice in you.
>
> Psalm 5:11

I vividly recall the first time I saw Frank Peretti's book *This Present Darkness*. I was in the small Christian bookstore situated as a side store to a large secular bookstore and located about three blocks from my house. As I stood in the glow of the fluorescent lights overhead, I stopped and stared at the ominous cover. A dark clawlike presence hovering over a tiny, steepled church beside blue water and against an explosive horizon. Captivated and standing transfixed, I was hardly aware of the salesgirl who'd stepped up to my right, poised to do her job.

When it comes to protection from the elements, author and speaker Jill Krieger Swanson (*Simply Beautiful Inside and Out*) says, "I use Revlon's Colorstay foundation, which has SPF 15. Honestly, as I've gotten older I find I have to take more pains to cover my face from the sun than ever before, particularly my eyes. I chose black-tinted sunglasses because they are the best for shielding out the light. Often I'll wear a hat. Because I'm very prone to getting cold sores around my mouth and nose, I never go without a lip balm with a strong SPF in it (Blistex Ultra Protection SPF of 30). But you have to read the packaging. Many lead you to believe there is an SPF when all it says is that it 'protects you from . . .'

"We deal with a dry, cold wind in Minnesota in the winter months, so a heavy moisturizer is a must. My product of choice is Vanicream or Eucerin Cream. They're found in drugstores and do the best job to moisturize all over. Far better than the expensive ones I've tried."

"What is it?" I asked. "It looks downright scary."

She took the book off the top shelf and said, "It's the latest in Christian fiction. And it's good. It's really, really good. If you don't have time to sit and read for a while, I'd advise waiting until you do, because once you pick it up . . . But, by all means, you *want* this book!" Presumptuous but correct, she handed the book to me.

I bought the book and—against the advice given to me earlier—began reading as soon as I got home. For the next long while I carried the book with me everywhere I went, devouring each word, forever reminded that there is a world out there that, although we cannot see it, exists nonetheless.

One of my favorite biblical stories is told in 2 Kings 6. Elisha, the great student of Elijah and a prophet in his own right, was with his servant in Dothan, which was located on a hill north of Samaria. In those days, about eight hundred years or so before Christ, Samaria was the place of the main royal residences of Israel.

Israel was at war with Aram. No matter what the king of Aram thought to do against the king of Israel, God would tell Elisha about it, and Elisha in turn would go and tell the king of Israel. The Bible tells us that "time and again Elisha warned the king, so that he was on his guard in such places" (2 Kings 6:10).

Naturally the king of Aram got suspicious and began to accuse his own men of treason. I'm not sure how it is that some of the men knew about Elisha and his relationship with God, but they did, and so they told the king, "Elisha, the prophet who is in Israel, tells the king of Israel the very words you speak in your bedroom" (2 Kings 6:12).

With no other recourse, the king of Aram determined that the only way to attack the king of Israel was by capturing the prophet who kept warning him. And so he sent orders to bring Elisha in. That night the army went to Dothan and surrounded the city.

The next morning, when Elisha's servant woke up and went outside to do whatever it is that servants do early in the day, he saw the army full of horses and chariots. Well, the man panicked. He ran to Elisha and asked, "What shall we do?"

Elisha didn't panic. Elisha prayed . . . more than just that God would deliver them from evil, but that the servant would be able to see that "those who are with us are more than those who are with them. . . . O Lord, open his eyes so he may see."

When the servant's "eyes" were opened, he saw that the hills surrounding them were filled with horses and chariots of fire, all of which surrounded Elisha. A heavenly host was on guard around the man of God, a heavenly host that mere humans could not see with their eyes but who, even so, were there.

King David (before he was the great king of Israel and while he was running for his life from his father-in-law, Saul) wrote, "The angel of the Lord encamps around those who fear him, and he delivers them" (Ps. 34:7). David understood that in times of personal threat, God would send his heavenly warriors down to protect his children.

The author of Psalm 91, who wrote that most poetic beginning—"He who dwells in the shelter of the Most High will rest in the shadow of the Almighty"—continued in his song with this promise: "If you make the Most High your dwelling—even the Lord, who is my refuge—then no harm will befall you, no disaster will come near your tent. For he will command his angels concerning you to guard you in all your ways; they will lift you up in their hands, so that you will not strike your foot against a stone" (Ps. 91:9–12).

Jesus, in speaking of his love for children, warned those who might look down on one of them that "their angels in heaven always see the face of my Father in heaven" (Matt. 18:10). When he was arrested, Jesus made a bold statement to Peter (who'd just cut off the ear of the Roman soldier Malchus) when he said, "Do you think I cannot call on my Father, and he will at once put at my disposal more than twelve legions of angels?" (Matt. 26:53).

These giants of our faith—as well as so many others—believed that something supernatural protects us, within reach and yet out of our ability to see. Question is, protects us from what?

When we're outdoors, playing or working in the hot sun, we are at war with an enemy we cannot see. We are not aware of UV rays until we see the damage they've done. That harm could come instantly in the form of sunburn or even a tan, which is actually brought about by damaging the epidermis. Or, the damage could take years to develop, as is the case with skin cancer or wrinkles.

The same is true when it comes to our spiritual skin. When we're "in the world," we find ourselves at war with an enemy we can't always see. Yet, the enemy is there. Listen to what Paul wrote to the church at Ephesus:

> Put on the full armor of God so that you can take your stand against the devil's schemes. For our struggle is not against flesh and blood, but against the rulers, against the authorities, against the powers of this dark world and against the spiritual forces of evil in the heavenly realms.
>
> Ephesians 6:11–12

That noted, I suppose you could say that the "full armor of God" is high SPF in your spiritual foundation.

In his description of the armor of God, Paul includes several things.

The Belt of Truth Buckled around Your Waist

The gospel of Christ is the belt of truth. But, how well do you know it? Recently the Bible study group I lead watched *The Gospel According to Matthew*, which stars Bruce Marchiano and Richard Kiley and is—in my humble opinion—the best Bible story movie ever made! As we watched the movie we also read from the book of Matthew while I handed out interesting facts along the way. What surprised me most as I prepared the lessons was my discovery of how *little* I—a Bible teacher and seminary graduate—knew the man, Jesus. Know the gospel! It's your best weapon of defense!

The Breastplate of Righteousness

In the ancient Middle East, a soldier's breastplate was made of iron and was fashioned in such a way as to protect the body from the neck to the middle and on both sides. Figuratively, our spiritual breastplate of righteousness wraps around us, protecting us from the arrows of our enemy. Righteousness has been cleverly defined as "right relationship with God," and in essence that means we are living a life that is holy and acceptable to God. The opposite of this term, I think, is "live by the sword, die by the sword."

Feet Shod with the Readiness That Comes from the Gospel of Peace

Just as those in the military are prepared to march, so should we be. Our "shoes" or "sandals" come from having both heard and understood the gospel of peace. Paul called it a peace that passes all understanding. In the midst of battle, we are at peace because we serve the Prince of Peace.

The Shield of Faith

Hebrews 11 begins, "Now faith is being sure of what we hope for and certain of what we do not see. This is what the ancients were commended for." It's amazing what we can endure when our shield is up. "Enemy, no matter what, I believe . . . I believe." That may be scary to even think about saying, but raise that shield anyway. Nothing but nothing can get through it.

The Helmet of Salvation

When my granddaughter was learning to ride a bike, I learned that scary times call for drastic measures. Bike helmets are now the law . . . and perhaps they should have always been. Knowing and being assured of one's salvation protects our minds from believing the lies of the devil.

The Sword of the Spirit

The sword of the Spirit, Paul goes on to say, is the Word of God. Remember when Jesus was tempted in the wilderness? What weapon did he have against the devil? The very Word of God. As Satan threw false prompting at him, Jesus merely quoted Scripture. Satan, in return, had no choice but to leave . . . to flee, as James puts it. "Resist the devil, and he will flee from you" (James 4:7).

Prayer in the Spirit

Though the last method of defense mentioned by Paul in the Ephesians reference, prayer nonetheless holds high importance. In John Gill's *Exposition of the Bible* he wrote,

> The last weapon is prayer, and takes in all sorts of prayer, mental and vocal, public and private; and every branch of it, as deprecation of evils, petitions for good things, and thanksgiving for mercies: and which should be used

Bonnie Engstrom, a homemaker from Southern California, says, "I started using Olay Complete Defense Daily UV Moisturizer with SPF 30 for sensitive skin last summer when I had to spend a lot of time in Arizona. It's creamy yet quickly absorbed and provides a smooth base for my makeup."

always: this stands opposed to such who pray not at all, or who have prayed, but have left it off; or who pray only in distress, and it suggests, that a man should pray as often as he has an opportunity; and particularly, that he should make use of it in times of darkness, desertion, and temptation: and this, when performed aright, is performed "in the Spirit"; with the heart, soul, and spirit engaged in it; it is put up with a true heart, and a right spirit, and without hypocrisy; in a spiritual way, and with fervency, and under the influence, and by the assistance of the Spirit of God.[3]

Questions for Personal Reflection or Group Study

1. Do you use a sunblock or sunscreen when you're in the sun? What SPF do you typically use?
2. Do you use a type of foundation or moisturizer with an SPF? If yes, can you see a difference in your skin? If no, why not?
3. How often do you "apply the whole armor of God"?
4. Why is it important that we daily do this?
5. Can you think of a time when you had applied the armor of God and were distinctly aware of the difference it made? What about a time when you felt you'd gone out unprotected? What happened?

Here's a Valuable Tip

There are no safe rays from the sun. None. Zero. Zip. Even a short period of time in the great outdoors and even cool or cloudy days can cause serious sun damage. As women—whether we are outside for pleasure or for work—we must consider the protection of our skin to be of the utmost importance. If you must be outdoors, try to avoid the hours when the sun is at its most blistering (noon to three). Apply sunblock and apply it often. When choosing the best product for you, be sure to read the back label and look for the following ingredients: zinc oxide, titanium dioxide, and parsol (avobenzone). These help block out UVA rays.

7

Skin Exfoliation

I consider that our present sufferings are not worth comparing with the glory that will be revealed in us.

Romans 8:18

Until I was in my thirties I had absolutely no idea what exfoliation was. Not even a clue. So right now, if you have no idea, fret not. Your time has come.

For me it happened like this: one afternoon I decided to go visit a friend. This particular friend was in her thirties and still single (at the time). She had a very good income and was able to pamper herself in ways I'd yet to know about. When I arrived, she greeted me with her engaging smile and twinkling eyes. That, and a cup of delicious and exotic hot coffee.

We sat at her stylish kitchen table for a while, talking about this and that, until she said, "Hey! I've got to get some cleaning done."

Now, I knew my friend had a maid that came once a week, and I couldn't imagine the damage one lone female could do in the interim. When my brow shot up, she added, "Closets and stuff. Come with me." She smiled as

> When it comes to skin exfoliation, Sue Sumser, a product merchandiser for Edy's Ice Cream from Winter Springs, Florida, says, "I keep a tube of Avon's Becoming Buff It Up! Exfoliating Body Polish in my shower. When I have time—about two to three times a week—I use it. I like the way it keeps my skin soft and also takes care of the dryness."

she grabbed me by the hand and dragged me down through the spacious rooms of her home, down the wide hallway, and into her master bath. Coffee mug still in hand, I sat on the tub's edge while she sat on the floor, legs crossed, with the under-the-sink cabinet doors opened wide and her head stuck deep within its caverns. We continued to talk (though her words sounded a bit muffled), and then suddenly my headless/armless pal withdrew her whole torso, holding up a half-filled clear tube with large green writing on it. "You ever tried this?" she asked.

"Tried what?" I asked.

"It's an exfoliation cream. Good stuff."

I narrowed my eyes, wondering what in the world an exfoliation cream was. My life had been filled with Jell-O and Play-Doh and a nice bar of Ivory soap. "No," I answered. "I haven't."

She threw the tube at me, and I caught it easily. "Here you go," she said. "Try this and tell me how wonderful your skin feels afterward. I've got tons of it."

The Body Beautiful—Physical

Therefore, if anyone is in Christ, he is a new creation; the old has gone, the new has come!

2 Corinthians 5:17

My lifestyle of regular exfoliation began with one try. After my first scrub (performed in the shower), my skin took on a healthy radiance. It felt smooth to the touch and younger somehow. As if the old me had been washed off my body and had gone down the drain.

"But doesn't skin naturally slough off?" you ask.

Yes, but it's a slow process, and one you would typically be unaware of. Your body is crying out for assistance in this, and the call must be reckoned. "Off with those dead cells," it shouts. "I wanna glow!"

"And what about showers? Or baths? Don't they do the trick?"

Nope. They're good for getting the dirt but do nothing for the "dead zone."

> Skin is the largest organ of elimination.
> Reference: About.com

Exfoliating your skin allows your newer (translate: healthier) skin to rise to the surface. Take center stage, so to speak, leaving a girl to look younger without having invasive surgery or, somehow, turning back the hands of time. It also cleans out pores clogged by makeup, the elements, or your skin's oils.

Skin exfoliation is beneficial to women of nearly every skin type. Women with oily skin may think the worst part about their skin type is having to pat their faces dry periodically throughout the day, having that shiny appearance, or even dealing with occasional or frequent acne. Not true. There is a more "invisible" problem. Oily skin tends to hold on to dead skin cells, keeping them from falling off as quickly as they ordinarily would. Women with dry skin have a similar problem: dry skin builds up dead skin cells too quickly, giving the skin an "aged" look. And who wants that?

Another enemy we face every day is, quite simply, nature's elements. Heat. Cold. Wind. Any and all of it places wear upon our faces. Boo-hiss!

While some people have exfoliation done professionally (either because they can afford to or because of medical conditions such as acne), you can do it easily at home, unless you have ultrasensitive skin, thin skin (from age), or some form of skin condition. The results will be healthier, smoother skin; an increase in its ability to absorb moisture, its muscle tone, and its new cell growth; and a reduction in those wonderful fine lines we find distinguishing on a man but aging on a woman.

> ### AT-HOME EXFOLIATION: WHAT YOU WILL NEED
>
> A soft washcloth; exfoliation mitt (such as nylon gloves) or brush, buff puff, or loofah; and the scrub of your choice. Look for those with round beads rather than rough granules, as the former is gentler on the skin.
> Or, if you are so inclined, you may purchase an at-home exfoliation system.

Skin exfoliation should never be rough. (I'd advise not doing it when you are angry about something.) It shouldn't hurt, though there might be some very mild irritation. (I can honestly say I've never had a bad experience with it.) You don't need a lot of product, either. For your face, the size of a quarter will do. Obviously you need more for the rest of your body. Before you start, be sure to use a gentle soap. When you are done, your skin will have a radiance even the sun couldn't have applied.

Chemical Peels

Some women, distraught over fine lines and wrinkles or acne, choose to have a chemical peel. Chemical (alphahydroxy acids or AHA) peels improve and smooth the texture of the facial skin by removing its damaged outer layers. They are performed, typically, by a plastic surgeon. There are states that do not require a medical degree, but personally, if someone were applying chemicals to my face, I'd want to see a medical degree, matted and nicely framed, preferably hanging somewhere prominent in his or her office. Before having a chemical peel, you should research both the procedure and the location of the procedure very carefully.

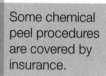

Some chemical peel procedures are covered by insurance.

Microdermabrasion

Microdermabrasion is a type of skin exfoliation using tiny crystals to remove dead skin. The results are the reduction of fine lines, wrinkles, small acne scars, and skin pores. Microdermabrasion also helps to improve skin color or dull, thickened skin.

Microdermabrasion uses an abrasive crystal (natural mineral) that is sprayed on the face (after a thorough cleansing) at a very high speed and then vacuumed back up. The procedure takes about fifteen to thirty minutes, and, although there may be some redness, salon or medical clients can usually put their makeup on and return to their normal daily activities, such as work or other social functions, without a telltale sign.

The Body Beautiful—Spiritual

You were taught, with regard to your former way of life, to put off your old self, which is being corrupted by its deceitful desires; to be made new in the attitude of your

Nancy Stafford, actress and Christian speaker and author (*Beauty by the Book and The Wonder of His Love*), has sensitive skin, so when it comes to exfoliation, she must be careful about what she uses. She says, "I only use a scrub when I'm really flaky and my skin feels rough and looks dull. Then, I use Francis Denny's Sweep Away for Sensitive Skin."

minds; and to put on the new self, created to be like God in true righteousness and holiness.

Ephesians 4:22–24

Have you ever sung the old hymn that went like this: "Are you washed in the blood, in the soul cleansing blood of the Lamb?"[1] If you spent any time at all in church as a youngster or at a rip-roaring, soul-claiming revival on a warm summer's night (fanning yourself with handheld funeral-home fans), then you probably have. It's a terrific song, reminding us that the blood of Jesus can "wash us" to a purified white.

The miraculous thing about being washed in the blood of the Lamb is that all the old sins that at one time covered our souls in filth are forever washed away. Sadly, however, this is not to say we cannot commit new sin, or that we suddenly become sinless. On the contrary. As Christians we must constantly rid ourselves of old habits, much like the old dead cells that want to build up on our physical bodies.

In the New American Standard Bible, Ephesians 4:17 and the section of Scripture that follows are headed as "The Christian's Walk." The NIV heads it with "Living as Children of Light," and the New King James Version titles it "The New Man." Interesting titles, especially considering that Paul focuses on those things that occur when we live the sinner's life, live as children of darkness, and live as the old man. In this passage, Paul warns against those things that will cause us to build up that old, dead skin that causes us to lose our luster and glow. "Putting off the old self," he calls it. For example:

- Do not live like a pagan, in futility of thinking. It causes a darkening of understanding, a life separated from God, and a hardening of the heart.
- Do not give yourself over to sensuality and indulge in impurities.
- Do not lie against your neighbor (which is anyone we come into contact with, especially on a continual basis).
- Do not let the sun go down on your anger.
- Do not give the devil a foothold.
- Do not steal.
- Do not talk "unwholesomely."
- Do not grieve the Holy Spirit.
- Get rid of bitterness, rage and anger, brawling and slander, as well as every form of malice.

In the midst of this, he gives us a few positive notations, reminding us that we have been created to be like God: truly righteous and holy.

- Put off the old self, put on the new self.
- Be made new in the attitudes of your minds.
- Speak truthfully to your neighbor (see above for definition).
- Do something useful with your hands.

- Share with those in need.
- Use words to build up one another.
- Be kind and compassionate to one another.
- Forgive one another, just as Christ forgave.

Wowser! Put those two lists together, and you've got one nice spiritual exfoliation.

When one reads the first list, it becomes quite evident as to why the "old" appears "ugly." Who wants to give off the appearance of being malicious, a gossip, or a thief? And who in their right mind would want someone saying, "You know [insert name here]? She sure is the most unwholesome person I've ever known. And what a *dark* personality! When it comes to her mind, it's garbage in, garbage out."

It's just so much prettier to think of someone saying, "What a beautiful woman of God [insert your name here] is!"

It's true. Just as skin dies or becomes calloused and hardened, so too do the hearts of those who do not get rid of the old and take on the new. Our previous lives are ugly to look at, certainly ugly to remember.

But, Paul essentially says that you decided you didn't want to live this way. You decided you wanted to exfoliate! Read these words again: "You were taught, with regard to your former way of life, *to put off your old self,* which is being corrupted by its deceitful desires."

Notice that Paul wrote "which *is* being corrupted." Is. Not was. Is. Even as believers, we can be easily influenced by the world's elements to become hard again. The end result is that we find our spiritual skin needing a good exfoliation.

No, we are not immune from temptation. Living in the world (not of the world but in it), we attract so many of its impurities.

In Colossians 3, Paul wrote another list of "rules for holy living." Within them, we see the method of spiritual exfoliation. In those verses we read that we are to set our minds on things above, not on earthly things, and put to death (exfoliate!) whatever belongs to our earthly natures. Examples Paul gives are sexual immorality, impurity, lust, evil desires, and greed, which is idolatry. In 3:9–10 Paul reiterates a common theme: "You have *taken off your old self* with its practices and have put on the new self, which is being renewed in knowledge in the image of its Creator" (emphasis mine).

The story of Lazarus of Bethany and his "four days in a cave" experience can teach us a bit about spiritual exfoliation as well. Lazarus was a friend of Jesus. In fact, Scripture tells us that Jesus loved Lazarus, so we can assume that they were the best of friends. When Jesus and his disciples had gone back to the place where John the Baptist had been baptizing in the early days of Jesus' ministry, they received word from Lazarus's sisters, Mary and Martha, that he was very ill. Rather than go back to Bethany immediately, he waited two days and *then* said, "Let's go back."

When Jesus and his disciples arrived, Jesus went to the cave where Lazarus's body had been entombed for, by this time, four days. He prayed to his Father in heaven, then called Lazarus by name. By the power of the Holy Spirit, Lazarus came walking out of the cave, bound by what were known as grave clothes.

"Take off the grave clothes and let him go," Jesus said.

The next chapter in the book of John gives us the last glimpse of Lazarus. He is sitting at the table, reclining with Jesus—who is not only his Creator but also his *re*-Creator! If Lazarus were dining with Jesus, then he was no doubt talking and laughing and—in general—having a wonderful

Erin Valentine, a homemaker from Bentonville, Arkansas, says, "I use Oil of Olay microdermabrasion twice a week, plus I use their Reginerist product at night before bed. I'm not nearly as well preserved as my little sister (who has never sunbathed because of a sun allergy), but people usually guess that I'm five to eight years younger than my actual years. So, I guess it's working."

time. The man probably had a special "glow" about him. After all, Jesus had just commanded life back into him and then demanded that his grave clothes be removed.

Talk about removing the dead and replacing it with the new! In the remaining years of Lazarus's life, what a testimony his very presence in a room must have proclaimed!

There's nothing better than being "scrubbed clean" by taking on the person of Christ. By being in his Word, lifting up praise and worship to his name, and making determined decisions to live as children of the light, we become renewed. The Holy Spirit gently takes away all those "nasties" we seem to attract, scrubbing us until we are fresh and clean and feeling renewed once again! Being one with Christ, we *glow*!

Questions for Personal Reflection or Group Study

1. Do you exfoliate your skin? How often?
2. How does physical exfoliation make your skin feel?
3. In what ways can you, personally, spiritually exfoliate?

4. Take a look at the lists Paul gives. What areas of your spiritual body need exfoliating the most?

5. How do you feel after having been "scrubbed clean" by the Lord?

Here's a Valuable Tip

You don't have to go to a professional for a chemical peel. There are lots of them on the market now, including those from at-home purchase companies like Avon and at drugstores and department stores. Just be certain that a chemical peel is for you and to follow the directions to the letter.

8

MOISTURIZER

Before a girl's turn came to go in to King Xerxes, she had to complete twelve months of beauty treatments prescribed for the women, six months with oil of myrrh and six with perfumes and cosmetics.

Esther 2:12

When I was a young girl, a woman with beautiful skin told me that if I would begin moisturizing at my present age, my skin would remain supple and smooth for years to come. "Don't wait until the wrinkles begin or your skin starts to stretch and itch from dryness," she said. "Then it's too late. Start now."

Thus began my love affair with moisturizing. Ironically, years later when I told my Filipino neighbor that I was expecting a child, she shared with me a little secret she'd brought to America from her mother and her mother's mother. "Keep baby oil on your stomach and hips," she advised, "and you won't have stretch marks." I did and I don't. Not a single one, in spite of the fact that I gained enough weight to cause my OB/GYN (and my mother) to become concerned.

Rebeca Seitz, president and founder of Glass Road Public Relations, from Fulton, Kentucky, says, "I use Arbonne Moisturizer as my body moisturizer. It has all-natural ingredients, and it works! Makes my skin look like a teenager's again!"

As if that were not enough to make me a believer, another incident sealed the deal. As a woman in my early thirties, I sat in a beauty salon next to an exquisite older woman. As her beautician styled her hair, she said, "It's remarkable to me that you are the age you are. Your skin just doesn't have the texture of a woman in her eighties." I looked over from my chair. The hairdresser was correct. Her skin was lovely. "What's your secret?" I asked.

"As soon as I'm out of the bath or shower," she said, "I pat dry—never rub—and then I immediately apply moisturizer. The wetness of my skin will soak in the lotion, thus allowing it to work more effectively."

That night, immediately following my shower and a patting dry of my skin, I began to apply moisturizer (aka body lotion) to moist skin. I've been repeating this ever since, and the results have truly been remarkable.

The Body Beautiful—Physical

> All beautiful you are, my darling;
> there is no flaw in you.
>
> Song of Songs 4:7

Allow me to begin this section by setting a couple of things straight. First, when we talk about moisturizing in this chapter, we're not talking about facial, hand, or foot lotion per se. We *are* talking about overall body lotion, body butter, and body cream in general. Second, too often we apply face or hand cream and forget about the rest of our bodies. That wrong is about to be righted.

And now for another clarification: regardless of the fact that moisturizer has the word *moisture* in it, these lotions do not put moisture in your skin. The point of a moisturizer is to help *hold* nature's oils and moisture in your skin. Naturally, the drier your skin, the less it has to work with, so it's important that you drink plenty of water to moisturize from the inside rather than simply from the outside.

As I said earlier, it's not uncommon for women to use moisturizer on their face and sometimes on their neck, but often they stop there. It is just as common to hear men say they don't use any moisturizer at all. (But, we're really not here to talk about them, are we?) Everyone thinks to use hand lotion when their hands are dry, cracked, or calloused, but how many stop to apply lotion anywhere else? Body lotion for your legs, arms, and torso is just as important as applying it to that part of your body that could launch a thousand ships.

> Whether you use moisturizers or not, the absolute best thing you can do for your skin is to drink plenty of water.

When our foremothers wanted to moisturize their skin, they used a variety of homemade lotions. Today, we are (I suppose) blessed in that we can drive to the nearest drugstore or shopping mall and walk out with any number of moisturizing lotions. Scented or unscented. Light or heavy. With tiny little moisture beads or without. This skin type or that skin type. You name it, these stores have it. If you've visited stores like Bath & Body Works or the Body Shop, you know that not only do lotions come in a number of scents but also you can match them with candles and soaps too.

However, before you run in and just grab up the first moisturizer that smells good, it's important that you know your skin type. If your skin tends to break out, you'll want to stick to an oil-free moisturizer. Whether oily or dry, however, look for a product with an SPF of at least 15 and ingredients such as petrolatum (seals in your skin's natural moisture) and alphahydroxy acid (which helps slow the wrinkle process).

When looking for a body lotion, cream, or butter, be sure to note if it is water soluble. These types of lotions, creams, and butters will dissolve in water (i.e., your wash) so there will be no film or buildup on your clothes or bed linens.

If you tend to have sensitive skin, you'll want to hang back from lotions with ingredients added for scenting. If your skin is dry, you'll want a lotion with a little more oomph to it, something more along the lines of a body cream or body butter, which are richer in emollients and are better at holding moisture in.

When it comes to body moisturizers, Julie-Allyson Ieron, author of *Praying Like Jesus*, says, "I use Ahava Dead Sea moisturizers. A friend brought them back from Israel last year—and I'm hooked! I had been having trouble with really dry skin—cracking, etc. I'm on the brink of turning forty, and everything about my body seems to be changing! Nothing I could find brought any relief, but Ahava is really working to bring back the youthful softness."

If you are in doubt at all about the best lotion for your skin type, your best bet is to hop in your car and drive to a local store or specialty shop so that you can spend some time talking to a trained salesperson.

The Body Beautiful—Spiritual

> I am gentle and humble in heart, and you will find rest for your souls.
>
> Matthew 11:29

The point of body lotions is to keep your skin soft, toned, and supple. Like our human bodies, our spiritual bodies should be kept the same. Looking and feeling good spiritually doesn't come about by a one-time-only application. The younger you start taking care of yourself spiritually, the better off you'll be later in life. This doesn't mean that if you come to the Lord at an older age, you're doomed. But, let's face it: you're more apt to be "scarred."

I am reminded of one of the many afternoons my grandmother and I would spend sitting in front porch rockers, swaying back and forth and talking about all the things in life a child of the sixties found important. One afternoon a neighbor of Grandmother's walked by and said hello. Grandmother talked to this woman for a few moments, and then the nice lady was on her way.

"What a sweet lady," Grandmother said.

I pondered that comment for a moment. I'd heard others say the same thing about Grandmother, a woman I admired to the nth degree. "You know what, Grandmother?" I informed her. "I've decided that when I grow up, I want to be a sweet old lady."

"How do you think you should go about accomplishing that?" my grandmother asked.

"I'm not really sure," I said with a shake of my head. "But I do know that you're a sweet old lady." (My grandmother graciously allowed me to live after this statement.) "How'd you get to be that way?" I asked.

Grandmother smiled knowingly. "Sweet *old* ladies," she instructed, "come from sweet *young* ladies."

Those words are so grounded in truth, they've stayed with me all these years. The way we treat our bodies now will be reflected—most typically—by the condition of our bodies when we are older. Likewise, the things we learn spiritually as children often keep us spiritually healthier as we grow older. Solomon wrote, "Remember your Creator in the days of your youth, before the days of trouble come and the years approach when you will say, 'I find no pleasure in them'" (Eccles. 12:1).

I heard a story once that so beautifully illustrates this point. It's the story of an elderly woman who, as she approached the end of her days on earth, began to lose the ability to speak and reason. As time marched relentlessly forward, she spoke less and less yet always managed to say her favorite words of Scripture, words she'd learned as a child in Sunday school: "He who began a good work in you will carry it on to completion until the day of Christ Jesus" (Phil. 1:6).

Time went on as, day after day, the woman stayed in the care of the nursing facility where she'd been living. After a while, the nurses and other medical personnel noticed that the only words coming from her lips were those from God's Holy Book. It soon became evident, however, that even those were slipping from their beloved patient's memory.

"He who began a good work in you will carry it on to completion," she repeated over and over, leaving off the last few words, "until the day of Christ Jesus."

Then: "He who began a good work in you . . ." she would say.

A few weeks later: "He who began . . . he who began . . . he who began . . ." she'd repeat.

Finally, the only words she said were, "He . . ."

As she slipped from this life to eternity with the *him* of her utterance, she was surrounded by family and the nursing home personnel who listened as she continuously whispered, "He . . . he . . . he . . ."

At the end of her life, her last words spoken reflected the One she'd loved and adored her entire life. From sweet young lady to sweet old lady.

How can we—any of us—keep our spiritual bodies soft, toned, and pliable? How can we age gracefully from sweet young ladies to sweet old ladies, no matter what our age may be at this time?

> But we have the mind of Christ.
> 1 Corinthians 2:16

We must begin by taking on the mind of Christ.

But, how do we, with all our sinfulness and worldly clutter—those things destined to damage our souls as the elements of nature can so easily damage our bodies—manage to take on the mind of Christ? The answer is so unbelievably simple and is as easy as applying moisturizer on a daily basis. We take on the mind of Christ by spending time with him. *Applying* him, so to speak.

Have you ever noticed that the more time you spend with someone, the more like them you become? I know this is so very true for me. I'm very quick to "take on" mannerisms, phrases, and even accents.

Years ago I had a friend named Melissa. Melissa was undoubtedly one of the sweetest people I've ever known.

Her voice was soft and gentle. Almost soothing, I'd have to say. I never, ever heard her yell or scream, even when she was miffed.

She was funny too. Very few things coming from her mouth weren't amusing to me in some way.

One time Melissa and I spent a long weekend together. Within a matter of hours, I began speaking more softly (my voice tends to be a bit harsh at times, but I don't mean to sound "mean" or anything!), and soon I noticed that I felt very calm. Peaceful. It was an emotion I quickly tuned in to and came to like, but one that went by the wayside just as fast when Melissa and I parted company.

Likewise, the more time we spend with the Lord, the more like him we become. It only goes to reason then that the less time we spend with him, the less like him we become. By reading the Word and praying continuously, we literally and liberally apply him to ourselves. Because he is the living water, our spiritual skin is able to "drink him in." He, in turn, can go deep into that part of us that may have gotten wrinkled, dry, or calloused.

Just as it is important to determine the right kind of body lotion for your skin type, so should you be sure that the "spiritual lotion" you are using is appropriate for you.

I was speaking to an old friend the other day. We'd not spoken in some time (he and his family had moved), and I asked what he'd been up to, where he was working, how his family was doing . . . things like that. At some point he shared with me that—after years of absence in his faith— he'd come back to the Lord. I told him how excited I was to hear it and then asked where he was attending church.

He shared the name of the church, followed by, "I just love it there, Eva. I love the teaching. It's the basic kind of stuff that I need to hear right now. It's seeker driven. And the music . . . oh, I could listen to the music all day, every day."

For my old friend, a seeker-driven church was just what he needed at this point in his spiritual walk. But someone who is more mature in their faith would certainly look for those things that would help strengthen their faith based on its current depth. I know folks who love a more contemporary worship service, as well as those who think that when the electronic instruments are brought out and the music is upbeat, they've landed just this side of Hades.

We must all find houses of worship that are the best fit for us. This by no means suggests that you should attend a church that doesn't challenge you or doesn't stay true to God's Word. Every believer—I believe—should find fellowship within a solid, Bible-based church where they can learn about the deep things of God. It's just that not every church community is for everybody. Some like choirs, and others like praise and worship teams. Some like a variety of instruments while others say, "Piano or organ only." Some like pastors in robes, and others prefer preachers in Birkenstocks. But always—*always*—make certain your church teaches biblical truths and is a place where you can grow spiritually.

Just as we should apply moisturizer every day rather than once a week or even every few days, so too should we daily spend time with Christ, and thereby take on his mind—and this means doing more than simply attending church once a week, or even a few times a week. Spending time with him includes spending time in his Word and in prayer. And—this is where my soapbox comes in—getting to know the One who has been from the beginning, and shall always be, means learning about his presence in the Old Testament as well as the New.

Terri Gillespie, the director of donor relations and development of Messianic Jewish Alliance of America, from Lansdowne, Pennsylvania, says, "Moisturizing-schmoisturizing, I've got the secret to a creamy body, and it ain't in a jar! It's fish oil, honey, Islandic Cod Liver oil. But, if you have visions of slimy fish goo, fear not, it's a pill. It'll do more for your skin (and joints, I might add) than Elizabeth Arden . . . although it's not as much fun."

Spending time with Christ means becoming spiritually in tune to his Spirit. When this happens, we begin to produce the fruit of the Spirit: love, joy, peace, patience, kindness, goodness, faithfulness, gentleness, and self-control. All those things mark us as "sweet ladies," whether young or old. How much better to carry those traits from the day of our youth by beginning this type of spiritual care early on, rather than later.

Questions for Personal Reflection or Group Study

1. What kind of body lotion do you use? Is it truly appropriate for your skin?
2. When did you begin using body lotions and moisturizers? If you had started younger (or later) in life, do you think it would have made a difference?
3. When did you come to know Christ? Were you a "sweet young lady" or did you come to know him as an adult? (If so, how might getting to know him earlier have changed your life?)
4. How spiritually supple are you? Would your family, friends, co-workers, and neighbors think of you were they to read about the fruit of the Spirit?

5. What does it mean to you to "take on the mind of Christ"? Do you think you have? If not, what would it take for you to do so?

6. What kind of church do you attend (I'm not asking denomination)? Do you feel you are being spiritually "moisturized" there? If so, how? If not, why not?

Here's a Valuable Tip

If you suffer from dry skin, exfoliate and then moisturize. Dead skin has a very hard time holding on to the moisturizers you place on your skin. If your skin appears "dull," try increasing your vitamin D. Foods rich in vitamin D are dairy products, egg yolks, and fish.

9

THE FACE

Now Laban had two daughters; the name of the older was Leah, and the name of the younger was Rachel. . . . Rachel was lovely in form, and beautiful.

Genesis 29:16–17

Who *doesn't* want to be beautiful? I mean, really? Who looks in the mirror and says, "I wish I were ugly"?

And what woman who has seen more than her fair share of sunrises and sunsets would not jump up, run out, and head for the nearest department store should she be told of a miracle in a jar?

Recently, while speaking at a conference and rooming with my good friend Janice, I sat in our hotel room, relaxing at the end of another grueling day, and flipped through a ladies magazine. There I read an article about a company and a product called La Mer. According to the claims of quite a few movie stars, this stuff is truly a phenomenon. Relatively expensive, but a phenomenon.

I had to know more. I went to my laptop and began to search the Internet. Moments later, I knew more about the product, and I knew where to find it. Fortunately (or, unfortunately, according to how you look at it) for me, one of the exclusive stores that offered the product just happened to be right across the street.

Before my unsuspecting roommate could say, "But I'm beautiful as I am," she was being whisked out of the room and bribed with dinner, and then was gliding down a second-floor escalator toward the inviting gleam of overladen cosmetic counters.

We were met by a lovely salesclerk, and I asked about the aforementioned product. She spoke to us knowledgeably, then opened the tester jar and allowed us to sample a bit of the cream by dabbing it with our fingertips and then rubbing it onto the backs of our hands.

It was fabulous, and we told her so.

"But," said the salesperson, "this is not really for you. You need to try this product over here." She guided us to the Orlane Paris counter, where two women stood in wait.

I asked about their line of product (after all, I was writing this book and needed the information) and was amazed by their depth of knowledge. One of the salesclerks in particular—an absolutely beautiful woman from Poland who also happened to be a district representative and an aesthetician—suddenly turned to Janice and said, "But of course you know what problem your skin has, don't you?"

Janice—who looked a bit like the deer caught in the headlights—declared that she did *not* know that her skin had a problem. For the second time in a matter of a couple of hours, she was being whisked away, this time to a nearby bar chair. The other salesclerk continued to talk with me, and out of the corner of my eye I could see Janice's makeup being removed and then not one but two Orlane Paris representatives working on her.

Minutes later I heard her exclaim, "Oh my gosh, Eva! You have no idea how wonderful my face feels right now!"

I looked over and saw my friend glowing. Just glowing!

I demanded my own makeover. (After all, I was the one writing the book!) Minutes later, I felt transformed. Truly. I could feel the difference even before I could see it in the nearby mirror. Again and out of the corner of my eye, I saw Janice, this time making a purchase. *Egad!*

Next thing I knew, I heard "What would you suggest for me?" coming out of my mouth. Then I swallowed. "And how much will it cost me?"

The salesclerk reached for a business card and began to scribble numbers on its back. She then slid it across the glass countertop as though we were haggling over the price of a car.

I looked down and . . . son of a gun . . . we *could* be talking about the price of a car.

Okay, a very broken-down one, but a car nonetheless.

To make a long story just a tad longer, I will tell you that I awoke the next morning in a dead panic. Had I really spent that much money on face products? But . . . a month later—having said nothing to any of my friends (partly because I

Karen T. Fahel, a part-time administrator for a financial advisory company and a full-time mom from Manchester, New Hampshire, says, "For my face care, I love to use Neutrogena or Clean & Clear, both liquid and scrub. At forty-one, I still haven't outgrown my adult acne. Neutrogena and Clean & Clear have been the most effective at keeping my skin at least tolerably viewable. Currently I am using Bioré, a product line my sister gave me for Christmas."

didn't want to hear about starving children in third world countries[1])—I had received a great number of compliments about how much younger I was looking these days. New haircut? Had I changed my hair color yet again? Then one of my more savvy friends said, "I don't know what new regimen you are using on your face, but it is working."

(Blush) and thank you. But, tell that to my budget.

The Body Beautiful—Physical

> My lover spoke and said to me,
> "Arise, my darling,
> my beautiful one, and come with me."
>
> Song of Songs 2:10

Yes, we all like to look pretty. While we know we cannot possibly keep the complexion of our twenties (and who in their right mind wants the blemish-prone look of our teens?), we'd at least like to think we could age gracefully. We look to the examples of movie stars and friends or family members who have done it and done it well, and we wonder what their secret might be.

My mother recently shared with me that she read an article stating you should always wash your face twice, beginning the process with warm water and finishing with splashes of cool water. She then said she remembered her aunt Mary Beth had always washed her face twice.

Aunt Mary Beth, at eighty-five or so years of age, continues to have one of the most remarkably beautiful faces a woman could hope for. But is washing the face twice the only right thing to do?

Most of us, unknowingly, are our own worst enemy when it comes to our faces. We spend too much time in the sun, unprotected. We scrub our faces as though we're cleaning glass, and apply makeup and moisturizer as though we're refinishing furniture. It's insane!

I'll tell you what else is insane: the contradictions you'll find in beauty books. Moisturize, one says. Don't moisturize, another says. Moisturize only if you have dry skin. Use only products with *this* ingredient. Avoid *that* ingredient. Never wear makeup to bed. It won't hurt if you wear makeup to bed as long as you washed your face somewhere between morning and bedtime. Retinol A is A-OK! Retinol A is AB-solutely unnecessary for a beautiful face.

Good golly. How's a girl to know for sure?

I don't want to add to the angst, so let me just talk about what I have learned along the way. (And I say these things as a woman who is often being told I look younger than I am, a compliment I'll take any day of the week and at any time of the day.)

If you don't want your face to betray your age or if you'd at least like to be considered beautiful at any age, you'll first want a clear understanding of the face's number one telltale sign of aging: wrinkles. To understand, you'll need to know what causes wrinkles.

It's pretty simple, actually. Muscle contractions. Years of smiling and frowning and making other facial expressions a caboodle of times. The website for Facial Plastic Surgery, Houston, Texas, has the following additional information:

> Wrinkles are a byproduct of the aging process. With age, skin cells divide slower, and the inner layer called the dermis, begins to thin. The network of elastin and collagen fibers, which support the outer layer, loosens and unravels, which results in depressions on the surface. With aging, skin also loses its elasticity, is less able to retain

moisture, oil-secreting glands are less efficient and the skin is slower to heal. All of these contribute to the development of wrinkles.[2]

Other factors leading to wrinkles are gravity, exposure to the sun and other damaging elements from Mother Nature (who, as a woman, really *should* be on our side), and excessive abuses to the body such as drugs, alcohol, and smoking. (The chemicals involved in smoking cause an increase in the aging process, not to mention what scrunching up your lips every time you draw on the cigarette does to your mouth.)

Now, you may be wondering, *What if I stop smiling (or frowning) and making other facial expressions? Can I prevent wrinkles?*

Probably not. Mainly because wrinkles also have to do with other factors, such as exposure to the elements and gravity. So keep smiling (avoid the frown) and think of other things you can do to help slow down the process (because you cannot stop it).

My guess is that your first thought here is to moisturize. Well, here's the bad news: moisturizing will not prevent wrinkles. However—and here's the good news—it *will* help wrinkled skin look less so. Dry skin just naturally looks older.

Though our ancestral sisters would use egg whites as a mask, vinegar for tightening the skin, rosewater for refreshing, and glycerin for moisturizing, today we are faced (pardon the pun) with a plethora of choices when it comes to fighting wrinkles. Everything from Botox to cosmetic surgery, AHAs to BHAs (alpha hydroxy acids and beta hydroxy acids), Preparation H to clay masks, and everything else in between.

Ultimately the products you choose will depend on what works for you and your pocketbook; this is not to say that the most expensive products out there are necessarily the best. It truly has to be about what works for *you*.

So, product names aside, let's just take a quick ten-point course I like to call "Facing Facts."

Facing Facts 1: When applying moisturizer, youth serums, or foundation, do not pull the skin or rub in a circular motion. Rather, use gentle, outward motions, which help lift the face.

Facing Facts 2: Day moisturizers should include a sunblock. Nighttime moisturizers should be a bit heavier, as the skin's absorption increases during this time.

Facing Facts 3: Remove your makeup with a gentle cleanser, again using outward motions. (And, by the way, always wash your hands before you wash your face or apply product.) When you are finished washing, pat—never wipe—your skin dry.

Facing Facts 4: Toners are an extra cleansing step that also leaves the skin refreshed. You'll want to find one that's alcohol free.

Facing Facts 5: Exfoliate once a week to once a month, according to your skin type (the more dry, the less you need to exfoliate). Same goes for skin masks.

> The only way to get rid of blackheads once you have them is to squeeze them out; they do not often get up and leave on their own.
> Paula Begoun,
> *Don't Go to the Cosmetic Counter without Me*

Facing Facts 6: One of the best things you can do for your outward look begins inward. Drink plenty of water, eat a healthy diet, and take necessary vitamin supplements.

Facing Facts 7: Keep your hands off your face so you don't pull or poke the fragile skin.

When it comes to facial care, former model, speaker, and author of *Beauty Quest*, Tonya Ruiz says, "I use Oil of Olay moisturizer. I've used it for twenty-five years. My daughter, an aesthetician, says I have beautiful skin. But my makeup drawer is a smorgasbord of colorful delights. Neutrogena foundation, Mary Kay blush and lipstick, and MAC eye shadows. One thing I remember from my modeling days is that if you notice the makeup instead of the face, you're applying it wrong. Makeup is supposed to accentuate features, not dominate them. Most women would benefit from a trip to a cosmetic counter to have their makeup done professionally. The makeup artists will write down what you need and how you need to do it. You can purchase there or you can shop at some other place, like a drugstore."

Facing Facts 8: Your face doesn't stop at your neck; it goes down your neck and on to your décolletage. It is vitally important you moisturize these areas as well. When doing so, use downward motions rather than outward.

Facing Facts 9: As we get older we have to deal with a nasty little thing known as facial hair. Again, you have choices: pluck them, bleach them, remove them with hair remover or waxing, electrolysis, or laser hair removal.

Facing Facts 10: If you wear foundation, remember: you should never, ever look as though you do. Foundation should blend exactly with your skin color and tone and should not appear to stop at the throat. You can help avoid this by applying it closer to your nose and then—using a sponge or brush—bringing it outward.

The Body Beautiful—Spiritual

> When Moses came down from Mount Sinai with the two tablets of the Testimony in his hands, he was not aware that his face was radiant because he had spoken with the LORD.
>
> Exodus 34:29

These are the words that follow one of my favorite sections of the Scriptures. Moses has led the Israelites from the clutches of slavery in Egypt. They are on their way to a new life in the land of milk and honey. Moses, as a man with whom the Lord speaks "face to face, as a man speaks with his friend" (Exod. 33:11), has spent much time with the Lord within what is known as the Tent of Meeting (Exod. 33:7). When Moses would enter the tent, the Word says, the pillar of cloud (a symbol of God's presence) would hover at the entrance of the tent. The people would be in such awe of this; they would worship at the entrance of their own tents from where they'd been watching.

During a particular chitchat with God not long after the wandering Israelites had sinned by creating the golden calf (see Exodus 32), Moses entreated the Almighty One to reveal even more of himself.

He said, "If you are pleased with me, teach me your ways so I may know you and continue to find favor with you" (Exod. 33:13).

He asked, "What else will distinguish me and your people from all the other people on the face of the earth?" (v. 16).

He pled, "Now show me your glory" (v. 18).

God sent Moses to a place on the mountain where he could stand "on a rock" and the glory of God would pass by. When this happened, the Lord said, he would place Moses in a cleft of that mountain and would place his hand over him to ensure that Moses did not see his face.

Before Moses experienced this magnificent moment, he chiseled out two stone tablets to replace the ones he'd broken when he'd seen the golden calf and gotten a bit miffed at the Israelites. Job complete, he then went up Mount Sinai.

> Then the LORD came down in the cloud and stood there with him and proclaimed his name, the LORD. And he passed in front of Moses, proclaiming, "The LORD, the LORD, the compassionate and gracious God, slow to anger, abounding in love and faithfulness, maintaining love to thousands, and forgiving wickedness, rebellion and sin."
>
> Exodus 34:5–7

Having presented his glorious self to Moses, God then wrote by his own hand what we call the Ten Commandments. Forty days and forty nights passed. In that time Moses neither ate nor drank; he spent intense and intimate time with God.

The result?

> When Moses came down from Mount Sinai with the two tablets of the Testimony in his hands, he was not aware that his face was radiant because he had spoken with the LORD.
>
> Exodus 34:29

This story is much like one that happened thousands of years later. Jesus, having climbed a high mountain (most likely Mt. Hermon, though traditionally it is said to have been Mt. Tabor), is transfigured just before having a little chitchat with Moses, who represented the Law, and Elijah, who represented the Prophets. Jesus was not alone on the mountain; Peter, James, and John had accompanied him and witnessed the event.

Matthew 17:2 reads, "There he was transfigured before them. His face shone like the sun and his clothes became as white as the light."

The three men observing this watched their beloved Christ as he conversed with Moses and Elijah. Then a bright cloud came down, and from the cloud a voice said, "This is my Son, whom I love." The boys were so knocked over they fell facedown. Later, Peter wrote these words: "We did not follow cleverly invented stories when we told you about the power and coming of our Lord Jesus Christ, but we were eyewitnesses of his majesty" (2 Peter 1:16).

> The word *transfigured* is *metamorfoo* in Greek. We get the word *metamorphosis* from the Greek word, which gives us the sense of divine radiance.

I have a friend who, though she'd gone to church since infancy, did not know the Lord. She said the blessing before meals, sang in the choir, and never missed a Sunday service unless she was sick or out of town. She was married and had a daughter she adored. Her job was fulfilling, and her home was lovely. Everything seemed to be perfect in her life.

But whenever I saw her, she always appeared to be just a tad on the unhappy side. The smile from her lips never quite reached her eyes.

Then, one day I received a phone call from her. She sounded absolutely exuberant. "I gave my life to Jesus!" she nearly screamed.

I stammered a bit. "I thought you already were a Christian."

"Oh, I lived life as a Christian. But I hardly knew Jesus," she said. "I'd never truly given my life to him. Now I have!"

She went on to tell me that she was going to take a few of her vacation days and go away for some time alone with him. "I'm calling it my honeymoon," she said with a laugh.

And, off she went.

Two weeks later I saw her for the first time since the phone call, and I hardly recognized her. Her face was . . . *radiant!* In fact, I'd have to say it was akin to the face of a woman in love. Perhaps in love with her Bridegroom, with whom she had just had a "honeymoon."

> My heart says of you, "Seek his face!" Your face, LORD, I will seek.
> Psalm 27:8

> I have chosen the way of truth; I have set my heart on your laws.
> Psalm 119:30

What happens when we "seek the face" of God, as David wrote in Psalm 27? What happens to our own faces—whether literally or figuratively—when we spend time with him, sharing with him, speaking to him, and listening for his voice?

Years ago I realized just how much of an Egypt I was living in. In spite of being a Christian, I had become immersed in the muck and the mire of my own sin. Then, one evening, I fell facedown upon my bed and cried out to the Lord. "I want to know *all* of you," I prayed. "I'm not afraid of anything you might show me."

It was the beginning of a new life for me. It didn't take long for others to notice that something was different, new. But if I wanted to keep this new look, I had to continue in the same type of care regimen that the physical face requires. (In other words, what if I washed or toned or exfoliated or moisturized my face only once?)

I had to spend time "in the tent of meeting." Let me rephrase that: I *have* to spend time in the "tent of meeting." I must worship the One who knows me best and yet loves me most; I must cry out, "Teach me your ways . . . so I might know you!"

Before Moses went up the mountain, he chiseled out the stones on which God's laws would be written. Our hearts are the new stones. We must bring them to God in our hands, ready for him to write upon them his will for our lives. His will being first and foremost that we love him unreservedly, putting nothing and no one before him. Only then will we desire to be with him more, know him better, and love him more deeply.

Our faces will show the results of time with God, of having surrendered ourselves to him fully, and of loving him completely.

Questions for Personal Reflection or Group Study

1. Have you ever gone outside your budget for a line of face products?
2. Has a beauty tip been passed down to you from an older family member? What is it?
3. Do you follow a face-care regimen such as cleanser-toner-serum-moisturizer? Why or why not? If not, do you think it would make a difference?
4. Describe any "mountain glory" experience you may have had. Did it change your outward appearance?
5. What does it mean to you to "seek the face of God"?

Here's a Valuable Tip

When our ancestor sisters wanted to do something about their wrinkles, they didn't hitch up the horse and buggy

Eileen Key, a retired teacher from San Antonio, Texas, says, "I'm still a Cover Girl girl. I've used it forever. I like its texture and color (# 105 Ivory) against my skin. I feel I get adequate protection and coverage for a good price. Plus, it's available wherever I go, not just at a specialty store."

and head to the storefront mercantile. Instead they tied on their aprons and headed to the kitchen. An old remedy for face wrinkles was to mix two tablespoons fresh cream (which may have come from the family cow) with one teaspoon honey. Stir the two together well, apply to your face, and allow to dry. Remove with a gentle cleanser.

10

EYES, THE WINDOW TO THE SOUL

I will set before my eyes no vile thing.

Psalm 101:3

Everyone has at least one asset, and mine are my eyes. Well, at least they used to be. Now the skin is a bit more "pulled" and "saggy" than it was in my youth. Still, my eyes—large, almond shaped, and brown flecked with amber—remain among my assets.

I was six years old when I came down with a vicious case of measles. My mother kept me in a dark room for two straight weeks in hopes that the measles would not "settle in my eyes," but apparently they did anyway. By the following school year, I was wearing glasses, those horrid cat-shaped things someone actually thought were fashionable. Those were the days when "boys never make passes at girls who wear glasses" was a common slogan and the term "four eyes" could often be heard on American playgrounds.

Deb Haggerty, president of Positive Connection, Inc., of Orlando, Florida, says, "I love Chanel eye makeup remover because it is gentle, yet thorough, and is non-greasy/oily. Although a bit pricey, it lasts a long time and helps my eyes look their best!"

I hated my glasses. They were ruining my asset.

Then, at about fourteen, when I was nearly blind, stumbling about in those Coke-bottle look-alikes, the optometrist suggested contact lenses. "You'll get more menses with contact lenses," my mother said, chuckling at her own humor. Whatever, as soon as I popped those puppies in I was heading for the local drugstore in search of Maybelline.

Blue eye shadow was the rage; I bought a tube of it in a cream, which turned out to be useless. I also bought mascara, which if I remember correctly was Maybelline's Great Lash, a product I still use to this day. (Why mess with perfection?)

In time I learned how to highlight and shade.

From the spiritual standpoint, I also learned the importance of what I expose my "eye" to. What good are beautiful eyes if they drink in only the ugliness of life?

The Body Beautiful—Physical

Then Jehu went to Jezreel. When Jezebel heard about it, she painted her eyes, arranged her hair and looked out of a window.

2 Kings 9:30

Okay, I couldn't help myself. I just had to begin this section of the "eye chapter" with the verse that preceded

Jezebel's "help" out of a window and onto a fatally hard surface.

I suppose the message here is: if you're gonna get tossed, do it lookin' good!

Which brings me to my next point: on those days when you're going sans makeup, at least wear mascara! Stroking on a little mascara (and a touch of lip gloss) makes all the difference in the world, and you won't look like you're heading for the mortuary.

That said, applying eye makeup is the trickiest of all cosmetic feats. Do it right and you'll be admired for your natural beauty; do it incorrectly and you'll be thought a clown.

There are five areas you need to think on when it comes to eye makeup.

1. Eyeliner
2. Eye shadow
3. Mascara
4. Brows
5. Removal

Eyeliner comes in a plethora of choices: thin pencils or fat pencils. Liquid in a tube, liquid in a cute little inkwell. Automatic pencils, felt-tip pencils, and pencils that need sharpening. Pencils with sponges and pencils with matching shadow.

Between 1960 and 1974, we progressed from wearing heavy liquid liner that swept over the eyelid and ended in wings at the back of the eye, to wearing Twiggy lashes, which were pointy lines drawn vertically from the lower lashes, with false lashes worn on the lid. Then, somewhere around 1976, smudge pencils became the fashion. The smudge sticks were great; they were fast and convenient and, sad to say, did just what their name said they would do; they smudged all over the place. Smeared eye makeup was a definite problem.

Paula Begoun,
The Beauty Bible

135

How's a girl to choose?

As complicated as it sounds, it's not. First, ask yourself, "What is the look I'm going for?" and then you'll have a starting point. You may not even want the eyeliner look. As we grow older, we want to look less harsh, and liner can quickly age us. The older we get, the more of a natural look we should attempt, although that could actually take more makeup than less.

Whether you are young or "less young," a few rules always apply:

1. Unless you are a runway model and in some funky sort of photo shoot, don't line all the way across the lower lashes or near the tear ducts.
2. When lining under the eyes, start in the middle and move outward. If you line underneath the entire length of the eye, your eye will look smaller.
3. Though most people don't follow this rule, makeup artists, books, and cosmetic articles seem to agree that you should use a softer shade of your liner for under the eye.
4. Some books say that eyeliner follows eye shadow. Others say reverse the process. The question is, what is the look *you* are going for?

Eye Shadow

Eye shadow is the tricky part of wearing makeup. So often, women go for overkill and just end up looking silly.

Applying eye shadow is an effort in artistry. Years ago, my daughter—who is very talented in this area—asked if she could "make me up." When it came to my eyes, she would get just the right amount of shadow on the brush, blow at the brush as though it were too much, and then seemingly become Michelangelo. When she was done and I was turned toward the mirror, I was amazed at the look. This was so much more than just a stroke of shadow. This was shading, highlighting, and contouring.

In my opinion, the best way to learn how to apply shadows on your eyes is to march yourself to a trained professional at one of the numerous glass display cases at a local mall or shopping center. If there isn't a mall available to you, go online, to the library, or your favorite bookstore and check out the step-by-step directions. Remember, the shape of your eyes and tone of your skin will determine the shades you want to wear.

Finally, do *not* use sponge-tip applicators as they pull the delicate skin above the eye. As a good friend of mine once said to me, "The secret is in the brush!"

> ## TWO RULES OF THE BRUSH
>
> 1. Never have just one. Have at least two or three.
> 2. Brushes should never be bigger than the area of application.

Mascara

As stated previously, I wear the same mascara today as I wore in high school. As far as I'm concerned, it's simply the best. I've tried expensive lines and always go back to the number one bestselling mascara in the country.

Again, mascara is the one cosmetic you should always wear when leaving the house, even if you don't wear anything else. Nothing changes your look like brushing on some color and adding some length to your lashes.

When shopping for mascara, look for those with conditioners and those that claim they don't clump. (Whether they do or not you'll have to prove to yourself.) If you're going to wear mascara that clumps, you might as well not. Even naked eyes look better than "spider leg eyes."

Don't "pump" mascara before applying it. Pumping inserts air. If you think there's too much mascara on the brush, use a clean tissue to wipe it down a bit and then apply.

Mascara comes in a variety of shades, but typically you'll want to stick with something that keeps you looking natural and classic. If length is all you are after, go for clear mascara.

If your new tube of mascara seems dry, return it to the store. If you've had your mascara for a bit and you want to extend its life just a tad longer, add a little distilled water (obviously, this applies only to water-soluble mascara).

And now for the question everyone wants the answer to: waterproof or water soluble? For me, the answer is simple: water soluble. Anything else is a bugbear to get off at the end of the day (I don't care how wonderful the remover is) and just not worth yanking my lashes out over.

You might also choose to curl your lashes. There are a number of eyelash curlers out there, including those that heat up, which I think are marvelous. Whatever brand or style you choose, make sure there's a little pad at the end. Also, curl your lashes before you apply mascara, not after.

Brows

Okay, we've all seen them, those women who draw their brows on and end up looking like clowns. The application of brow pencil or powder takes an expert hand . . . or at the very least a steady one! But before you "draw," you'll want to pluck.

Actually, before you pluck, you'll want to draw.

Allow me to explain. It is my understanding that we all have a "masculine" and a "feminine" brow. (In other words, your brows are not identical to each other; one is more round while the other is more angular.) So, as you sit before that magnifying mirror, take a minute to study the natural shape of your brow. Next, begin this painful process by drawing the shape of brow you are going for. It's the shape of the brow that can totally change the look of your face. It's like the frame on a painting.

If you are unsure about the best shape for your face, the arch, the length, etc., go to someone who can help you, typically in any salon across America. In fact, I suggest that your first shaping be done by a professional with occasional trips back for waxing, and save the plucking for between visits.

When it comes to self-plucking, be sure you use good tweezers and a magnifying mirror. When you're done, brush the brow (in fact, you should brush your brow every

When it comes to her eyes, author and speaker Karen O'Connor (*Squeeze the Moment: Making the Most of Life's Gifts and Challenges*) says, "I remove eye makeup at night, rinse my eyes with a cleansing solution, pat dry, and always get plenty of sleep. If I feel eye strain from too many hours at the computer, I take a couple of five-minute 'eye naps' during the day. I lie on the floor, listen to music, and relax with my eyes closed. I also get regular eye checkups. Common sense and basic care have paid off. According to my doctor, I have excellent vision and eye health for a woman over sixty!"

day) with an eyebrow brush or a child's toothbrush, which is cheaper unless it's a character toothbrush (like Barbie or Superman), but that's another story.

Your brow pencil or shadow should match the color of your natural brow, not your hair color. Literally every book I've read says this, so it must be so.

The Body Beautiful—Spiritual

> Open my eyes that I may see
> wonderful things in your law.
>
> Psalm 119:18

It's been said in a number of ways.

Eyes are the mirrors of the soul.
The face is a picture of the mind as the eyes are its interpreter.
The eyes are the window to the soul.

Jesus said it this way: "The eye is the lamp of the body. If your eyes are good, your whole body will be full of light. But if your eyes are bad, your whole body will be full of darkness. If then the light within you is darkness, how great is that darkness!" (Matt. 6:22).

From the spiritual perspective, it was our eyes that got us into all this mess. Look at these verses from Genesis 3:

> Now the serpent was more crafty than any of the wild animals the LORD God had made. He said to the woman, "Did God really say, 'You must not eat from any tree in the garden'?"
> The woman said to the serpent, "We may eat fruit from the trees in the garden, but God did say, 'You must not eat

fruit from the tree that is in the middle of the garden, and you must not touch it, or you will die.'"

"You will not surely die," the serpent said to the woman. "For God knows that when you eat of it your *eyes* will be opened, and you will be like God, knowing good and evil."

When the woman *saw* that the fruit of the tree was good for food and pleasing to the eye, and also desirable for gaining wisdom, she took some and ate it. She also gave some to her husband, who was with her, and he ate it. Then the *eyes* of both of them were opened, and they realized they were naked; so they sewed fig leaves together and made coverings for themselves.

Genesis 3:1–7, emphasis mine

There has always been a correlation or connection between physical and spiritual eyes, and the "craftiest of all" knew this. If he can put something in front of our eyes that is luscious enough to cause desire, then he can begin to destroy us spiritually. This is why porn is so powerful. It's what we see with our eyes that stirs our sexuality (which is God's gift!) toward a far-from-godly end.

> I lift up my eyes to you, to you whose throne is in heaven.
>
> Psalm 123:1

Ah, but ladies! The same goes for jewelry, fashion, that adorable comforter set you just couldn't live without . . . anything!

It's interesting to me that the words of Jesus in Matthew immediately precede that famous verse, "No one can serve two masters. Either he will hate the one and love the other, or he will be devoted to the one and despise the other. You cannot serve both God and Money" (Matt. 6:24).

Years ago I made a decision to be more careful about what I read or watched. This choice followed a series of depressions I couldn't quite explain . . . until I realized that my days of sadness always followed the viewing of a particularly favorite movie (if I like a movie, I'll watch it to death!). This particular film, Roman Polanski's *Tess*, was a period piece based on a classic, *Tess of the d'Urbervilles*. It was filled with romance, passion (the good kind), and loads of angst. There was hunger, death, rape, and murder. The ending was not a happily-ever-after, but it was one that made my heart catch in my throat.

Some time later I became nearly addicted to romance novels. I read them ad nauseam. I had a composition book with a list of my favorite authors and a list of what I had read, and I'd even developed a rating system for each title. It always accompanied me to the used bookstore where the clerk and I were greeting each other on a first-name basis and practically exchanging recipes.

> There are six things the LORD hates, seven that are detestable to him: haughty eyes . . .
>
> Proverbs 6:16–17

All that to say, I can tell you from firsthand experience that at around page 220 of a romance novel the big passion scene takes place. Words like *loins* and *throbbing* and *violent shiver* can be found. The more I read (typically propped up in bed), the more I'd arch an eyebrow toward my adorable husband and wonder, *Now why can't you take me like His Grace just took Angelica?*

It was wrong. One evening in a fit of frustration, I hit my sleeping husband with the book I was holding and said, "If you men would read these books, we women wouldn't have to!"

It was to be the end of my secular romance novels days.

David wrote, "I will set before my eyes no vile thing."

In his masterpiece work *The Treasury of David*, Charles Spurgeon writes concerning this third verse of Psalm 101:

I will set no wicked thing before mine eyes. I will neither delight in it, aim at it or endure it. If I have wickedness brought before me by others I will turn away from it, I will not gaze upon it with pleasure. The psalmist is very sweeping in his resolve, he declines the least, the most reputable, the most customary form of evil—no wicked thing; not only shall it not dwell in his heart, but not even before his eyes, for what fascinates the eye is very apt to gain admission into the heart, even as Eve's apple first pleased her sight and then prevailed over her mind and hand.[1]

Not everything that is wicked appears to be so. I'm sure Eve's fruit looked perfectly innocent just hanging there on the tree, but it was forbidden. In our world today there seem to be so many things that appear innocuous at first sight but that are not, and many of us are left to wonder how we are to know.

It is by the gracious gift of the Holy Spirit within us that our spirits catch that "check" that says, "Turn away." The problem comes when we do not listen to that voice or act upon that check. Suddenly, like Eve, we are doing more than looking; we are touching, and then, like addicts drawn to a needle, we are biting into what at first appears to be luscious fruit but later turns sour in our stomachs.

> For the word of God is living and active. Sharper than any double-edged sword, it penetrates even to dividing soul and spirit, joints and marrow; it judges the thoughts and attitudes of the heart.
> Hebrews 4:12

Let's go back to David for a moment. While we can cheer him for such powerful words and strong conviction, we all know he failed miserably on that fateful evening when he peered down from the roof of his palace to the roof belonging to Uriah the Hittite and his wife, Bathsheba. What did he see? Bathsheba, bathing.

Nancy Williams, owner of Nestle Down Inn B&B from Stover, Missouri, says, "For pretty eyes, I use eyeliner and smoky mauve powder shadow with brown/black mascara. I use Signature Club A (Adrienne Arpel) and just play around with it myself until I get the look I want."

Did he turn away? No. He did the human thing; he continued to look.

But we are not called to stay within the boundaries of "humanness." When tempted, we are to pray or—as Jesus did in the desert—call upon the Word of God, which cuts sharper than a double-edged sword. (See Matthew 4; Hebrews 4.)

Like applying makeup to the eyes, it's not always easy. It takes practice. Sometimes you'll get it right. Sometimes, as with eyeliner, the line will get a bit shaky. But keep trying and trusting God, and you'll be sure to get it picture-perfect.

Questions for Personal Reflection or Group Study

1. How much makeup do you wear around your eyes? How does it change your look?
2. When you reflect on Eve standing before the Tree of the Knowledge of Good and Evil, how do you imagine her wrestling with the decision of partaking or turning away?
3. What measures do you take to make certain that "no wicked thing" is set before your eyes?
4. Can you think of a time when you felt the Holy Spirit "check" in your spirit, and you responded? What

about a time when you did not? What happened with each time?

Here's a Valuable Tip

One of the most daunting problems women have when it comes to their eyes is dark circles underneath. Well, don't feel alone in your struggle; it's a common malady caused by various factors from lack of sleep to heredity.

In an online article for AZCentral.com,[2] Lisa Kasanicky reports there are three ways to get rid of dark circles: camouflage (concealer or foundation, which must be properly applied to work), treat (under eye moisturizers), or correct (lightening agents).

She also reports these old methods are still used by the pros today:

- cosmetic cotton squares soaked in milk or witch hazel
- chilled cucumber slices
- cooled chamomile tea bags
- grated raw potatoes wrapped in cheesecloth

11

THE OLD KISSER

Whatever your lips utter you must be sure to do, because you made your vow freely to the LORD your God with your own mouth.

Deuteronomy 23:23

Do you know what a Cupid's bow is?

I mean, besides the little thingy Cupid uses to shoot his love arrows.

On the face, and particularly on the lips, it is the place where the upper lip curves or peaks to form what looks like an archer's bow. Not everyone has a Cupid's bow. I do and I love it. It's one of the things about me that I can look at and say, "And Eva saw that it was good."

But what I don't like so much are my teeth. In spite of the braces, they are still crooked, and my dentist says they are a "strange color." (They don't look that strange to me.) I have spent megabucks on caps and bridges and, yes, whitening. I've tried it all.

For years I had a slightly chipped front tooth. Most people said they didn't notice it, but it was the first thing I noticed

> Pam Meyers, a retired administrative assistant from Arlington Heights, Illinois, says, "For the past couple years I have used Cover Girl's Outlast Smoothwear. It comes in a package with liquid lip color in one container and the gloss applicator in another one. It lives up to its claims. I put it on in the morning, and I can go all day and still have some color on my lips when I go to bed that night. I don't have to remember to keep reapplying lipstick, which is something I have a problem doing. It doesn't come off when you kiss either! So you can be assured your guy won't have the lipstick on him."

in photographs and when I looked in the mirror. I practiced smiling in that mirror so the chip didn't show in photographs. (Had to do with the placement of my lower lip.) Then, last year, my new dentist (the same one who made the comment about the color of my teeth) did a quick little filing and voila! I no longer have a chipped tooth, slight or otherwise.

But the smile—which had been perfected—remains the same.

The Body Beautiful—Physical

> Set a guard over my mouth, O Lord;
>   keep watch over the door of my lips.
>
> Psalm 141:3

You know it's true. Our mouths can do so much for us. So much good. So much damage.

My husband and I have a friend who manages to drive us bats from time to time. (Okay, a lot of the time.) The things that come out of her mouth can quickly be misunderstood; it seems to be a plague with her. But when she smiles . . . you melt. You just *melt*.

There's more to a pretty smile, however, than wearing the right shade of lipstick or having near-perfect teeth. In fact, the mouth—such a tiny little member of the body—requires a lot of personal attention. Attention that begins behind the lips.

Your Teeth and Other Oral Issues

Never mind having pretty teeth. You want *healthy* teeth.

My friend Allison teases me because I spend so much time on my teeth. I told her, "You would too, if you'd had the problems with yours that I have had with mine." Because of childhood illnesses and the antibiotics I had to take, my teeth aren't a pearly shade of white. They were also prone to cavities. They were crooked and "bucked." Seems I was always in a dental chair; my permanent teeth literally glittered with silver! At twelve I got braces (though a few of my teeth ran right back to where they'd started from), which I wore for two painful years. This was, of course, followed by the retainer. Then, at about age fourteen there was an "unfortunate incident" with the hygienist, and I refused to go back. For years, I didn't go back. (I know . . . yuck.) What I did do, to compensate, was to brush, brush, brush. Brush and floss. Floss and brush. Mouthwash, mouthwash, mouthwash. Whatever the American Dental Association was recommending, I did. After eight years I had not one single cavity in my teeth.

Ah, but now I'm kissing fifty, and all those old fillings have turned against me. I now have crowns and bridges where teeth used to be, and they also came with a great deal

There are many different types of floss, most of which are available with or without a mint flavor:

- **Waxed** and **unwaxed floss** are the most common. Some people prefer waxed floss because it slips between the teeth more easily than unwaxed floss and is less likely to break.
- **Tape floss** is flat rather than round and is typically thicker than regular floss. Tape takes less force to get in between your teeth than the regular round type, so some people prefer it.
- **Super floss** is used to clean under bridges. It has a thin piece of floss that you feed under the bridge, which you then pull through until you reach a thicker piece. This thicker piece cleans under the bridge next to the gum line.
- A **flosette** is a plastic handle that holds a length of floss. It can be held in one hand and can make it easier to direct where the floss is going than using your fingers.

Published by BUPA's health information team, healthinfo@bupa.com, April 2005

of pain. I realize now just how precious teeth are. You need them for eating, and you need them for smiling!

When I was a little girl my mother had a friend whose front tooth was badly chipped. When she laughed, she covered her mouth with her fingertips. Years later, I had a family member (now living with Jesus) whose teeth just kept falling out. (She was in her late eighties and early nineties at the time.) By the time she died, she was gumming her food.

Our teeth come to us when we are but babies, and we want to keep them until the day we die. To do this we have to keep them healthy.

So how can you do this?

Brush them. Twice a day at a minimum. (I say, brush after you eat.) There is a wide variety of toothpastes out there, from fluoride to non-fluoride, whitening to sensitive. Find the best one for you and your needs. When it comes to your toothbrush, look for one that is small enough to reach all your teeth and has soft to medium bristles (which is best for the gums). Or, you may choose an electric toothbrush, which is better at removing plaque.

If you are a businesswoman, keep a small toothbrush and a traveler's tube of toothpaste in your purse or briefcase. Should you have a lunch meeting, after the meal excuse yourself and head to the ladies' room. (Finer restaurants have a decanter with mouthwash and stacks of small disposable cups just for this purpose.) Brush your teeth, powder your nose, and reapply your lipstick.

Let's say you aren't a businesswoman. You can still carry your oral cleaning supplies alongside your tube of lipstick and lip liner, and it doesn't have to be a bulky burden to you. Most drugstores have travel-size toothpaste and toothbrushes.

I cannot stress enough the importance of flossing. I read somewhere that brushing without flossing is like bathing only 65 percent of your body. Floss takes care of the bacteria that sneaks in between your teeth and escapes the bristles of your toothbrush. It also helps get rid of embarrassing bad breath (which we've all had at one time or another).

If you hate to floss, you may want to think about a Waterpik, which sends out a jet of water to clean between teeth and under the gum line.

Mouthwash is also important, and there are many to choose from. Each type of mouthwash does something different, so before you purchase, know what you are looking for. Fluoride mouthwash will help strengthen the teeth against decay. Total care mouthwash does the same and also freshens breath. Antiseptic mouthwash (who *hasn't* used Listerine?) will help kill mouth bacteria and freshen breath. Be careful, though. Antiseptic mouthwash has been known to stain teeth.

Lipstick, Lip Liner, and All the Other Products for Your Lips

The new thing these days is "lip plumping" lipsticks. Quite frankly, the last thing I want is to look like a bee stung the outside of my mouth. So, I've steered clear and can tell you nothing about them. But I could fill your ears and every single page with what I know about lipstick. If you'll be so indulgent, I'll fill you in on a tiny little secret.

> I have a good friend who says that when I die and am laid out beautifully in my satin-lined casket, she will walk by every so often and touch up my lipstick so I won't meet Jesus looking dead already. I know it makes no sense, but that's what she says, and I've made certain she has a tube of my favorite color, just in case.

[Whispering] *My natural lips look like I died about three months ago.* Seriously. They are truly a "whiter shade of pale." Because of this—and because I don't want to frighten folks—I've tried nearly every lipstick, lip gloss, and lip liner on the market. With the exception of one product[1] (which I'll buy from now until forever), no matter what I've tried, no matter how much I've spent, I always end up with the same dilemma; in a very short period of time, I look dead again. (Yes, I've tried the all-day/eight-hour miracle-in-a-tube, and they "travel" on me.)

All this said, I've learned a few tricks along the way.

1. Before purchasing, put a bit of the lipstick on the back of your hands. If it feels greasy, it won't stay on long, sorry. If the lipstick smeared as it went on, it won't stay long either.
2. Wear lip liner. (We'll talk about this more in a minute.) Do you remember coloring pretty princesses on

coloring book pages as a little girl? Do you remember when you learned to trace the lines in the color before shading in? The end result was a finished-looking princess. (Or frog or prince, etc.) The same goes for your lips. Line them first, and they'll not only look more finished, but also the color will last longer.

3. Put a tad of foundation on your lips first. Then the liner . . . then the lip color.
4. Another neat trick is to fill in your lips first with the lip liner, then color over your lips with your lipstick.
5. Using a lipstick brush versus applying the lipstick directly onto your lips helps keep the lipstick on longer. It also keeps you from putting on more lipstick than you need, which may eventually bleed anyway, and keeps the "clumps" away.
6. Lip gloss doesn't last. (It's also not something you want to wear in a professional setting but more in the evening, when you're doing something zany and fun, or when you are just so young you have no reason to care, nor should you!) A tiny bit of gloss over lipstick, however, makes for a nice look.
7. Before reapplying your lipstick, make sure the old is off. This keeps the new from falling into the cracks of the old.
8. Forget the old hint of blotting. Blotting removes lipstick. It doesn't seal it. If you want to seal it, place a tissue over your lips and lightly add loose powder.

Be sure to note the shade of your lipstick in relation to any colors worn close to the face, such as those in blouses, sweaters, and scarves. (You don't want the colors to contrast.)

When you apply lip liner, don't try to make thin lips look plumper or plump lines look thinner by way of the liner.

> Wearing a blouse that matches your lip color will bring a beautiful healthy glow to your face and a day filled with compliments. It is one of the most attractive colors you can choose for a top. When you are feeling under the weather, it will perk up your look and restore color to your cheeks. A shirt or sweater in your lipstick color is also an excellent option if you plan to get your picture taken.
>
> Jill Krieger Swanson,
> *Simply Beautiful*

That can be done with colors (thin lips look better with bright colors), and you won't look kinda funny or clownlike when the lip color wears off. When you apply lip liner, begin in the center of the upper lip and, using a light touch, head toward the corners of your lips. Avoid the absolute corner, though. Then go back to the center and head in the opposite direction. The bottom lip should begin at one end and go to the other. Again, keep your grip light and your strokes feathery.

I suggest talking to a professional about your best colors, but please note that your colors should change with the seasons. Something lighter for spring and summer and something darker for fall and winter. But make sure they are your best colors.

When it comes to her lips, author and speaker Carol Kent (*When I Lay My Isaac Down*) says, "I wear Perfect Peach by Merle Norman. This product has a lip liner on one end of a thick pencil and lipstick in my favorite shade on the other end. It stays on all day, and it's been my 'best pick' for over twenty years. Many companies don't sell colors that work well for redheads, so this product has been a winner for me, a woman with a fair complexion and auburn hair."

Finally, if you have "problem" lips, you might want to look at some lip-treatment products. Lip balms and creams are a worthwhile investment if you tend to have cracked or chapped lips and can help prevent those nasty lines we tend to get. Another tip (along those lines and mentioned previously) is to be careful of how much you purse your lips, especially to do something unhealthy like smoking.

The Body Beautiful—Spiritual

> With the tongue we praise our Lord and Father, and with it we curse men, who have been made in God's likeness. Out of the same mouth come praise and cursing. My brothers [sisters], this should not be.
>
> James 3:9–10

I could hardly believe the words I was hearing. Venomous. Filled with anger and bitterness. Words with complicated meanings meant to hurt the hearer. Line upon line of dialogue that was so enmeshed in rage, most of it didn't make sense.

Even more difficult for me was that I knew well the one speaking. In my lifetime I had come to both love and despise her. There were times I thought I knew her better than anyone else possibly could and other times I was certain I didn't know her at all. I'd seen her love people in spite of their faults, touch little children with tenderness, hold the dying as they took their last breaths. I'd heard her praising God, encouraging others, laughing at the joys of life. With all our ups and downs, I couldn't abandon her. Even now as she humiliated me with her words.

You see, she was me. I have to live with myself, even when I don't want to. Even when I allow my tongue to get the better of me.

155

"The tongue has the power of life and death, and those who love it will eat its fruit" (Prov. 18:21) says the proverb writer. The tongue can do so much good and yet yield so much damage. "He who guards his lips guards his life, but he who speaks rashly will come to ruin" (Prov. 13:3).

Two such powerful verses among so many others like them; you'd think we'd learn, but we don't. We talk and talk and talk and talk, and we rarely listen or contemplate. We're so accustomed to everything coming at us fast and going out just as hastily that we rarely slow down long enough to hear what is being said to us—*truly* being said to us—nor do we give enough time between what we hear and how we respond.

Sometimes we women—by our nature—just like to gab. Whatever is going on in our lives or is on our minds, we feel as though we have to tell somebody about it. There are times when some of us become so desperate, we'll grab a stranger (which is actually a fairly safe way to unload, given you'll probably never see the person again) if we have to.

But you know you've got a problem when your New Year's resolution is "talking less . . . listening more."

The tongue has the power. Power. Say it out loud: *power.* Can you begin to know what command you have within your very mouth? Words are powerful.

God created with words. "And God said . . ." we read time and again in the opening chapters of our beloved Bibles. Not that God "thought," but that he "said." Every word he spoke as a human—as Jesus the Messiah—is held in such reverence that we "red-letter" them. Pastors and writers and speakers have built sermons and articles and books on his last words spoken from the cross. Matthew considered his words of such value that he ended his Gospel letter with dialogue from the Master. And we who have come after men like Matthew and Mark and Luke and John, and women like the Marys and Martha and Lois and Eunice pray that we can be more like Jesus. In *word* and in deed.

The tongue has the power, but we should have control over the tongue. When we gain control, we will then determine whether good or bad—life or death—will be the result. We must note, however, that the proverb writer has given us a promise: those who love it will eat

> And whatever you do, whether in word or deed, do it all in the name of the Lord Jesus, giving thanks to God the Father through him.
> Colossians 3:17

its fruit (18:21). Delicious, satisfying fruit or rotten, rancid fruit; the choice is ours.

"But no man can tame the tongue," James wrote in his letter to the twelve tribes scattered among the nations (3:8). No man.

Or woman.

But, the Holy Spirit can. If "all things are possible" (Matt. 19:26) with God, then even taming the tongue should be. I believe—fervently believe—that this begins by reversing any negative purpose (on our part) for the tongue. To do this, you must go back one more step and realize that, though so tiny, it is so powerful. As James wrote, it only takes a bit to guide a horse and a rudder to control a massive ship (James 3:3–4), but there's *someone* controlling the bit and the rudder.

Understanding and accepting that though small, the tongue is powerful, we then turn it over to God. Begin this process by speaking praises to God rather than words to others. "With the tongue we praise our Lord and Father" (James 3:9).

One of my favorite things in my prayer time is giving God "praise offerings," especially in the midst of trials. As

I begin to "thank" him for the nasties of life, I am able to let go and allow him to take them and turn them into good. "And we know that in all things God works for the good of those who love him, who have been called according to his purpose" (Rom. 8:28).

From there I can move on to thanking him for all the good in my life, every little thing, right down to the glory of the sunrise and the food in my pantry, the health of my children, the provision and love of my husband, and my adorable grandchildren. The list here is nearly endless. Thanking God for the good in my life fills my heart with more good. Jesus said, "For out of the overflow of the heart the mouth speaks" (Matt. 12:34).

> My mother always said, "Cursing is an ignorant man's way of using the English language." I grew up never once hearing my parents use curse words. This made a huge impact on my life as a Christian and as a woman.
>
> Eva Marie Everson

As one who travels a good bit from church to church, speaking at women's retreats and conferences, I am always amazed at some of the words I hear, primarily coming from the lips of young Christian women. We seem to have adopted (or perhaps adapted) a lax way of speaking, including using swear words in our everyday language as casually as we would *and*, *but*, *for*, and *or*. Words that, in my youth, were considered vile coming from a young lady are now "acceptable," even in Christian society.

But, I wonder if they are okay for heavenly society. I wonder if our words might be more guarded if Jesus were walking beside us, dining with us, shopping with us, or having coffee at our kitchen table while we chatter nearby on the telephone.

Now, please don't think I have this down pat. There may be words I use (like *darn*, for example) that are displeasing to

Jeanne Marie Leach, an assistant innkeeper from Frisco, Colorado, says, "I have used Avon exclusively for makeup and skin-care products. I've tried many others, but I always come back to good old Avon. I've used Avon for over thirty-one years and receive many comments on how nice my skin looks—even from strangers! For lip dryness, I use Avon Moisture Therapy Lip Balm. I keep one on each level of my house and one in my purse for whenever my lips feel chapped."

my precious Lord. I pray, right now—with you, I hope—that the Holy Spirit will begin this very minute to put a check in my spirit whenever my words offend him.

Just as we take special care in oral hygiene, put balm on our lips, line our lips before applying color, and then look for the perfect lipstick, we must take great care when it comes to the words of our mouth. Pretty lips can draw eyes. Controlled words can draw ears. Speak goodness. Speak loveliness.

Speak Jesus.

Questions for Personal Reflection or Group Study

1. How careful are you when it comes to oral hygiene?
2. Have you had any corrective procedures done?
3. What's your favorite lip product?
4. Is your tongue in your control or the other way around?
5. How do you feel about swearing?
6. What plan of action can you design to help you gain control of your tongue?

Here's a Valuable Tip

When all else fails, there is also cosmetic dentistry, which includes:

- Whitening. There are a number of whitening procedures, both over-the-counter and dentist-supervised. Contact your dentist to find out which is best for you.
- Bonding. A solution for chipped or cracked teeth, bonding applies an enamel-like material to your damaged tooth, which is then sculpted and polished.
- Implants. Move over, dentures. Implants are stronger and more attractive, though most people I've talked to who have had implants stress the pain, so . . . you may want to have a long talk with your dentist before going this route.
- Veneers. Very popular process for those who desire the perfect smile. Veneers are custom-made laminates affixed to the teeth.

12

HANDS AND FEET

How beautiful on the mountains
  are the feet of those who bring good news,
who proclaim peace,
  who bring good tidings,
  who proclaim salvation,
who say to Zion,
  "Your God reigns!"

Isaiah 52:7

When it comes to my hands and feet, I have a love/hate relationship.

I hate my hands. I recently watched a tape of myself on a television show, and it left me frowning. When I see them in photographs (or on video), I want to call the "hand doctor" and beg for some sort of treatment. Or, if possible, a transplant. In turn, when I look at a particular family photograph—the one with my great-great-grandmother sitting stoically in front of my great-great-grandfather—I realize that my hands are part of my inheritance.

Not that I'm blaming Great-great-grandmother Mozelle or anything. That's just the way it is . . . or—in her case—

161

> Barbara Eubanks, a pastor's wife and retired teacher from Albertville, Alabama, says, "My biggest beauty luxury is going to Top Nails for regular manicures and pedicures. As a writer and humorist, I am before audiences and feel I should literally put my best foot forward. When I sign books, people do notice my well-manicured hands."

was. We have large hands, big knuckles, and showy veins. Fortunately for her, she lived in a time when women wore gloves upon leaving the house. Unfortunately for me, that's not in style today.

Now, when it comes to my feet, it's a different story. I actually love my feet. (Perhaps *love* is too strong a word. I *like* my feet.) My husband says I have the prettiest feet he's ever seen. Even though I've never been a big fan of wearing shoes (I was born and reared in the South, where children spend their summers running barefoot through the thick green grasses and along creek banks), and even though you can often see me walking down the sidewalk in front of my Florida home with unclad feet, and in spite of the fact that I've broken my little pinky toes so many times I've lost count (catching them on the corner of furniture while walking barefoot through my house), my feet have remained . . . pretty.

Maybe I should have been a foot model.

The Body Beautiful—Physical

I want men everywhere to lift up holy hands in prayer.

1 Timothy 2:8

Hands

"I would suggest," Florence Littauer said to me at her CLASS[1] conference, "that you get a manicure. You tend to use your hands when you speak . . . in fact, I'm not sure you *could* speak if you didn't have your hands."

I looked down at my nubby nails split and broken from constant use and abuse. "It's true," I said, nodding. "I use my hands when I speak." I let out a pent-up sigh. "And, you're right . . . they are not attractive."

When I arrived home, I called Sharon, who has a nail salon in my area. She said she could see me on Tuesday morning at nine. Since then, Sharon has been doing my nails every other Tuesday morning at nine. The old polish is removed, cuticles are pushed back, a thin layer of acrylic is applied, buffed, and then repolished. Of course, there may be more to it than that. And, to tell you the truth, Sharon is more like my therapist than my manicurist. Sitting there for an hour, I spill my heart and soul out while my hands are made more beautiful.

Well, in my case, less unattractive.

What I have discovered over the years of having my nails done is that whether you have inherited hands to die for or hands to cry over, and whether or not you choose to see a nail tech several times a year or not, caring for your hands is fairly basic but extremely important.

The hardest-working parts of our bodies are the hands and feet. When it comes to our hands, housework, gardening, and life in general put wear and tear on an often-neglected and always-exposed area. What began as soft and pliable ends up calloused, gnarled, and freckled with age spots.

So, what's a girl to do? For starters, consider investing in a paraffin wax treatment home spa. Paraffin (not a true wax but a waxy crystalline substance that in the pure form is white, odorless, and translucent) is not only wonderful for renewing dry skin but also acts as a hydrating treatment, perfect for sore muscles and arthritis. If you can't go that route, purchase a pair of gloves (yes, the old-fashioned kind) and nightly coat your hands in a thin veil of petroleum jelly. Then put the gloves on and go to bed. Within a short period of time your hands will feel absolutely wonderful and will look younger too.

Of course, hand lotion, ladies, hand lotion. Put a bottle of it everywhere! At your desk, next to the bathroom and kitchen sinks, at your vanity, and next to your bedside. Use it, and use it often. It doesn't have to be expensive, but you should want it to have some sort of moisture guard and be nongreasy.

When it comes to nail polish, be sure to use a color that is complementary to your coloring, clothes, lip color, and time of year. It's a lot to keep up with, I know, but think of how many times your hands get noticed. You want the experience to be good, no? However, if you think that expensive polish necessarily means the polish will stay on longer, this is just not true. The key is the formula of the polish, proper application, and what works best with your nails. You should also know that polish stays on acrylics longer than on natural nails.

The decision to wear fake nails is entirely up to your preference and your budget. Some fashion divas simply have "bad nails." I say that because I am one of them. I have had acrylics put on for years now, but I do occasionally give my nail beds a break and have them removed. If you prefer natural to fake but have brittle or thin nails, try one of any number of nail strengtheners on the market. Find the one that works best for you. (The one that worked beautifully

RULES OF THE
AT-HOME MANICURE

1. First things first: remove the old polish and remove it well. If you have natural nails, use nonacetone remover. While it's not gentle, it is less harsh.
2. File your nails with a file or emery board, using gentle strokes. Don't saw at them or scrape your nail bed.
3. Using nail scissors, trim the nails (if necessary). Do not trim to the quick.
4. Soak your hands in warm soapy water for just a few minutes to soften the cuticles. Finish by drying and applying cuticle cream.
5. Using a cuticle stick, gently push the cuticles back. Do not cut the cuticle. Wash and dry your hands.
6. Apply a base coat. Wait for it to dry for at least a minute before moving to the next step. If you want a clear coat only, you're done. If not, move to step 7.
7. Apply the first coat of your chosen color beginning at the side of the nail and then moving toward the center and on to the other side. This should be a one-two-three process.
8. Wait for the first coat to dry. This could take five to ten minutes. Be patient. Read a magazine. Make a phone call. But don't fold your warm laundry or attempt to pull a cake from the oven.
9. Apply the second and, if necessary, third coats of polish. Again, wait for them to dry before moving forward.
10. Apply a top coat. Top coats can be reapplied daily if so desired.

When it comes to hands and feet, author and speaker Julie Ann Barnhill (*Motherhood: The Guilt That Keeps on Giving*) says, "I'm a soft hands/soft heels at all cost type of gal. Slather on Vaseline and pull on a pair of socks and go to sleep. It is as (if not more) effective as expensive products on the market. Even at age forty and going barefoot as much as possible, I'm still smooth, smooth, smooth . . . my heels and hands, that is!"

for my daughter caused my nails to become more brittle, so again, it depends on *you*.)

Feet

I was attending a conference where it was acceptable to wear sandals. I'd never had a professional pedicure done before, but with my cute little summery outfits and adorable sandals, I felt it was necessary to plunge right in and get it done. Though the tech fussed at me for walking barefoot outside (she could tell by the roughness of the heels and balls of my feet) and I had to practically pinky-swear not to do it again (in spite of my feelings, which are that if we were supposed to wear shoes 24/7, we'd have all been born wearing a pair of Pradas), the experience as a whole left me so loving it, I called my mother and said, "You just *have* to do this!"

She refused, but that's another story.

When it comes to feet—you know, those things we walk on every single day, pretty much all day long—well, we just tend to ignore them, don't we? We stuff them into shoes that go against our foot's natural growth pattern, force them to carry all our weight merely on the balls, blister the bottoms of them by walking barefoot on hot cement or the heels of them by wearing too-tight shoes. Acts that are just as unhealthy as baking in a hot sun for hours for the sake of a tan or sucking on a cigarette for the sake of cool.

And then, to add insult to injury, we basically just ignore them. Sure, every so often we dash into a salon or day spa, and, dipping our tootsies into the warmth of the foaming water and relishing the moments they are being pampered by the nail tech, we think this one trip will undo years of damage.

Not so. Our feet need us, ladies, just as badly as we need them! So here are some basic tips for happy toes:

1. While showering or bathing, be sure to wash your feet well. Take time to give them a little extra attention.
2. While you might not use a foot scrub every single day, you should think about using one at least once a week. The circulation in your feet will be improved, and the skin will be nicely exfoliated.
3. Don't forget to do the same types of things to your toenail beds as you would your fingernail beds. Keep the nails nicely trimmed, rounded off at the ends, cuticles pushed back, nails buffed. Paint them if you'd like or simply apply a nice topcoat for shine.
4. About once or twice a week, use a file (designed just for the feet) or pumice stone for getting rid of the calloused areas.
5. As you would your hands, moisturize! Personally, I always enjoy applying a nice peppermint-scented foot lotion and then slipping my feet into some warm cotton socks or slippers.
6. If you suffer from "tired" feet, the next time someone asks you what you'd like for your birthday or Christmas, tell them an at-home foot spa. Especially

When it comes to pedicures, author and speaker Susan Titus Osborn (*A Special Kind of Love: For Those Who Love Children with Special Needs*) says: "One of the most relaxing things I do is go to my little local shop, Generation Nails, and get a pedicure. For five extra dollars they will massage my feet for ten minutes—for ten dollars I get a twenty-minute massage. That is a heavenly experience. In the summer I have flowers painted on my toenails. That becomes a wonderful conversation starter. I go every other week. It is a special time when I can sit back, relax, and be waited on hand and foot—literally."

if it's one of those things you just don't see buying for yourself (though I can't imagine why not!).

The Body Beautiful—Spiritual

Then Peter and John placed their hands on them, and they received the Holy Spirit.

Acts 8:17

Hands

Ah, the hand. So much has been said and written about it. It is with our hands that musical instruments are made and then played. It is with our hands that we greet each other. It is with our hands that we bless or comfort one another. With our hand we join the hand of another as we pledge our lives and love. What a beautiful picture.

The Scriptures also talk about the "work of the hands." Deuteronomy 14:28–29 says that by the works of our hands our blessings are poured out.

At the end of every three years, bring all the tithes of that year's produce and store it in your towns, so that the Levites (who have no allotment or inheritance of their own) and the aliens, the fatherless and the widows who live in your towns may come and eat and be satisfied, and so that the LORD your God may bless you in all the work of your hands.

When Jesus healed, he more often than not laid his hands upon the person (although it was not necessary). Luke 4:40 reads, "When the sun was setting, the people brought to Jesus all who had various kinds of sickness, and laying his hands on each one, he healed them." But Jesus also used his hands to bless people, especially children. Oh, how Jesus loves children!

Mark 10:16 says: "And he took the children in his arms, put his hands on them and blessed them."

In his second letter to Timothy, the apostle Paul wrote, "For this reason I remind you to fan into flame the gift of God, which is in you through the laying on of my hands" (2 Tim. 1:6). Paul had passed the gift (Greek *charisma*, which is divine grace, faith, holiness, virtue, knowledge, and/or the empowerment to serve Christ and his church) of God on to Timothy, a remarkable young man whose mother and grandmother were so noteworthy they were mentioned in Paul's letter to his "son." Timothy's spiritual strength was such that it carried him to his martyred death. But it began with a touch of someone's hands.

We lift up our hands when we give a benediction, or a blessing. From a priestly standpoint, this action began with Aaron. "Then Aaron lifted his hands toward the people and blessed them" (Lev. 9:22). Before his ascension, Jesus, our high priest, gave a blessing to his followers and disciples. "When he had led them out to the vicinity of Bethany, he lifted up his hands and blessed them" (Luke 24:50).

When we pray, we are commanded to "lift up holy hands." Paul, in his first letter to Timothy, said, "I want men everywhere to lift up holy hands in prayer, without anger or disputing" (1 Tim. 2:8). Did you catch the word before "hands"? Holy, Paul wrote. Holy hands. If we are to lift our God-given hands back toward their Creator, they should be—must be—"undefiled by sin, free from wickedness, religiously observing every moral obligation, pure, holy, pious."[2] I know of only one way to achieve this: we must constantly approach the throne of grace, asking of the Lord that he would forgive our sins—both intentional and unintentional. Otherwise, how can our holy God hear? "When you spread out your hands in prayer, I will hide my eyes from you; even if you offer many prayers, I will not listen. Your hands are full of blood" (Isa. 1:15).

Above all, whether my hands are lifted in prayer and praise or blessing another, I want to know that my hand is held firmly in the hand of God.

Years ago I was autographing books at a book buyers' convention. As the publisher's representative slid another copy of the book in front of me and a bookstore owner stepped before me, I did a quick read of the owner's badge. "You own a bookstore in Minnesota?" I said as a way to make small talk.

"Yes," he replied. "I do."

I began signing my name. "How's business up there in Minnesota?" I asked.

"It's been slow," he answered honestly.

For a reason I still cannot explain, I reached my hand toward his and clasped it. "Tell you what," I said. "Let's pray." We both closed our eyes as I lifted up these simple words: "Father, I pray you will bless the work of this man's hands as long as his hand holds on to yours."

We both said amen, he gave me a thank-you, then took his book and stepped away, allowing the next person, a woman, to step forward. Before I had a chance to say anything, the woman (another bookstore owner) reached for my hand. She wanted a prayer too! I repeated the prayer several hundred times that morning, and with each one I envisioned the bookstore owners, managers, and representatives extending their hand to our heavenly Father, clasping it, and then hand in hand working together over the course of the years. It was an awesome thought! *Our hand in his . . . our hands doing his work . . . his hands blessing our work, the work of our hands.*

What a wonderful thing is the human hand!

Feet

It was my most vivid nightmare.

My friend Robi and I had gone to the beach for a couple of days to sit and read and, in general, revive ourselves. On our first night there we snuggled down in our separate beds, chatted a bit about our lives and our ministries, and then turned off the light and went to sleep. A few hours later I awoke, sweat dripping from my body (yes, the air conditioner was on), shaking almost violently from the dream I'd just had. In it, I was traveling and in a ladies restroom. A prostitute (whose feet had been severed) attempted to "eat" my feet. Fangs exposed, she came hissing toward my legs as I screamed, "Noooooo!"

At that moment, I awoke. Not wanting to wake Robi, who slept peacefully across the room, I managed to make my way to the bathroom, where I flipped on the light, sank to the floor, and began to pray. Minutes later I "heard" a song in my head, over and over, that rang out, "How beautiful . . . how beautiful . . ." By the time I was back in my bed (with the bathroom light left on and the door cracked), the words had formed in my mind: "How beautiful are the feet of those who bring good news" (Rom. 10:15).

The next morning I told Robi about my dream. Mouth gaping, she said, "Well, it doesn't take a dream interpreter to figure *that* one out." We began to pray together daily about the path God was taking me down and the Good News I would be spreading in my ministry. We asked other prayer warriors to do the same.

Months later I was at a convention in—of all places—the same city I was in when I had my dream. Even though I wasn't looking for footless prostitutes, I was very much aware of Satan's desire to "stop my feet."

Then, on my last night, I returned to the hotel from dinner to discover that one of my roommates had left a "calling card" on my pillow. On one side were pictures of a variety of shoes. Victorian shoes. Sandals. Go-go boots. On the other were these words:

> How beautiful are the feet of them that preach the gospel of peace.
>
> Romans 10:15 KJV

In his beautiful way, God had reminded me of my calling and of his hand over that calling. He also told me that, to him, my feet are beautiful. But to Satan, my feet and the gospel of peace message they bring is an ill-fitting shoe!

Of course the "original" beautiful feet belonged to Jesus. His feet walked mile after mile, day after day, for three and a half extraordinary years, to tell humankind that God loved them. In a society of anything but peace, Jesus brought a message of internal, uncrushable peace. Our feet must follow in his footsteps.

A few years ago, while in Israel, I was walking up to the ruins of Bethsaida with five other journalists. Our guide turned to a layout of stones embedded in the earth and said, "These stones were a part of the original road and have been here for over two thousand years."

We were hot (it was June) and perhaps a bit tired. We looked at the stones and then back to the guide. "Ah," we said. Or, "Oh." Or, "Interesting."

The guide smiled. She could see from our expressions that we were clueless. "I said, these stones were a part of the original road and have been here for *over two thousand years.*"

A lightbulb went on over our heads. Eyes wide, we turned toward the stony path. Jesus had walked here. So narrow was the trail, surely his feet had graced every single one of the rocks. Before the guide could say, "And now as we move forward . . ." we were kneeling on the road, praying, asking the Lord to guide us and daily remind us that we follow in his footsteps, not the other way around. As he brought the Good News, so must we.

No matter the cost.

Just as we should care for our physical feet, we must care for our spiritual feet as well. Again, three words: *soak, smooth,* and *soften.*

Soak. One of the best things we can do for our physical feet is to rest them. Same goes for our spiritual feet. There are times we are called to rest. Even God rested, both on the Sabbath day and when he lived on earth as a man. As we rest, we allow God to repair us, thereby restoring us in our ministry—whatever that ministry is. Some of us are called to minister in the traditional sense; others are called to what I believe is an even higher call of ministry: raising children.

Smooth. Just as we slough away the calluses on our physical feet, so we must do so on our spiritual feet as well. What, in life, has made you "hard"? Bitterness can set in like a seed in fertile ground. Allowed to germinate, it will sprout like a weed and begin to choke out that which

Sandra Bishop, a freelance writer from Portland, Oregon, says, "The one thing I have figured out is that good foot care is a necessity for me. (And my hubby appreciates it when I take care of my feet.) Especially in the height of summer and winter when my heels crack like old porcelain and feel like sandpaper. At home, in between pedicures, I use Sally Hansen Smoothing Foot Cream—it's a paraffin-based product that helps roll off old skin and keeps my heels softer than they would be otherwise. I've heard that walking barefoot on carpet is terribly drying for feet, so I always wear socks in the house. In the winter I wear the fluffiest, softest ones I can find. In the summer, I keep several pair of flip-flops around to wear in the house. And, I never, ever go outside barefoot (except at the beach). I do splurge on pedicures occasionally, usually when we're on a trip, or just before. I usually pick one color of polish for each season, and just touch it up in between, with the same polish (which I buy from the salon). I have a caddy I've filled with the self-pedicure supplies, and I use porcelain nail files instead of emery boards."

is fruitful. It must be dealt with appropriately—be pulled out by the root.

Soften. As we massage away the cares of the world that seem to twist into knots in our feet—softening and soothing the skin in the process—we can do the same with our spiritual feet. Allowing someone to rub your feet is very intimate in nature. Allowing Jesus to "rub your feet" will lead to a deeper intimacy with him as well. Anoint them with time spent in God's holy Word. Soften them with prayer. Restore them completely as you engage in intimate moments . . . your feet in his lap, his hands applying his Word, his truth, his presence.

Questions for Personal Reflection or Group Study

1. How do you view your hands? When you look at them, do they remind you of your mother's or grandmother's hands?
2. How do you envision the hands of God?
3. When you pray, do you lift your hands? What do you think this symbolizes?
4. Read 1 Corinthians 12:21. Why do you think Paul specifically mentions the hands as a part of the body of Christ?
5. How hard are you on your physical feet? What about your spiritual feet?
6. Have you ever encountered a time when it seemed that Satan was trying to rob you of your ministry? Talk about it.
7. How much time do you spend "resting" in the Lord?
8. What anger, resentment, or bitterness has caused your spiritual feet to harden? What do you think you should do to alleviate this?

9. Close your eyes. Can you imagine Jesus massaging your feet? How can time spent in his Word and in prayer help to massage away the stresses in your spiritual feet?

Here's a Valuable Tip

For your nails to be healthy, your diet should include a lot of fruits and raw vegetables so that they get the required vitamins, minerals, and enzymes. Eat food that is rich in silicon like broccoli, fish, and onions. Eat foods rich in biotins like whole grains. Drink plenty of water and fruit juices. Food rich in zinc and vitamin B will strengthen your nails. Fresh carrot juice rich in calcium and phosphorous is perfect for strengthening nails. In addition, remember the following things:

- Lack of vitamin A and calcium in your body causes dryness and brittleness.
- Lack of protein, folic acid, and vitamin C causes hangnails.
- White bands across the nails are a result of protein deficiency.
- A lack of sufficient hydrochloric acid can cause splitting nails.
- Lack of vitamin B12 can lead to dryness, very rounded and curved ends, and darkening of nails.
- Insufficient zinc can cause development of white spots on the nails.[3]
- Cuts and cracks in the nails may indicate a need for more liquids.
- Red skin around your cuticles can be caused by poor metabolism of essential fatty acids.

13

FRAGRANCE

Pleasing is the fragrance of your perfumes;
your name is like perfume poured out.
No wonder the maidens love you!

Song of Songs 1:3

In my daily ritual of bathing (something those around me are grateful for), I do something known as "layering."

Layering is when you use scented bath soap or shower gel in your bath or shower, followed by patting dry and applying body lotion in the same fragrance, and then ending with a spritz or dab of the complementing body spray, cologne, or perfume. This results in an aura of the bouquet about you. Almost as though it comes from you naturally rather than from a shelf at the drugstore or a glass case at the department store.

What I love most about layering, however, is the lingering scent in our master bath, even hours after I've showered. I can shower and layer in the morning and not reenter the room until early afternoon, yet the bouquet of my favorite scent is still there. Reminding me of

> Sandy Bloomfield, a freelance editor and writer
> from Central Florida, says, "I like to blend Amarige
> by Givenchy with a dash of Happy by Clinique. The
> citrus scent of Happy would be too much without the
> Amarige."

something lovely. Something deliciously intoxicating and wonderful.

The sweetness of being a woman.

The Body Beautiful—Physical

> How delightful is your love, my sister, my bride!
> How much more pleasing is your love than wine,
> and the fragrance of your perfume than any spice!
>
> Song of Songs 4:10

Our sense of smell can evoke a wealth of emotion. When I smell coffee, I immediately think of cool mornings and being curled on a patio chair with a cup of my favorite drink, watching the sun peek over the eastern sky. Talking to God. Sharing in his wonder and majesty.

When I smell cinnamon I think of heart and home. When I smell Tabu, the classic fragrance by Dana, I remember my first "love," a young lad named Lonnie. Lonnie's mother wore Tabu, and the richness of it spilled over to everything around her. Including her son.

> When you leave a room there should be a hint of you that remains—your fragrance.
> Gale Hayman, *How Do I Look?*

It was her "signature" fragrance.

My author friend Jill Rigby layers her favorite fragrance, an inexpensive but fabulous product from Parfums de Coeur Body Fantasies. Last year, while we were together in a downtown Denver hotel, I stepped out of our room during her morning shower. When I came back about a half hour later, I said, "Mmmm. I smell Jill!" She laughed and said, "I'm such a creature of habit."

Not really, Jill. You simply have a signature fragrance; in this case, Fresh White Musk.

We all know that what smells wonderful on one person won't necessarily have the same scent on another. The chemical makeup of the bottled fragrance combined with our God-given scent will either set us apart or make us stinky. We want the former, not the latter.

In order to know what works best on you without spending a fortune, go to a department store or discount store and try the tester. However, note that what you smell when a fragrance first hits your skin is not what will remain. It will take anywhere from ten to fifteen minutes for that to happen. My suggestion is that you put it on, then walk around a bit. If you can walk outside in the fresh air, it will be helpful for making your decision.

Some of us prefer cologne to perfume. Others prefer body spray to eau de toilette. But what's the difference?

Four kinds of perfumes can be distinguished according to the quantity of oil they contain:

Parfum

Eau de parfum

Eau de toilette (toilet water—I know, sounds disgusting)

Eau de cologne

Most perfumes are complex combinations of natural materials, such as essential oils from plants, and synthetic products that increase the lasting power and heighten the smell. Alcohol, which allows the fragrance to go from your body to the nostrils of others, is used as a liquid base for perfume, and the ratio of alcohol to scented perfume concentrates determines what the final concoction is labeled.

From highest concentration to least, the different forms of perfume are:

- *Parfum,* also called *extract* or *extrait perfume,* can include 15–40 percent perfume concentrates. This is the purest form of scented product and is the most expensive as a result.

- *Eau de parfum* contains about 7–15 percent perfume concentrates. This is the most popular and common form of perfume. It provides a long-lasting fragrance and generally doesn't cost as much as extract perfume.

- *Eau de toilette* has around 1–6 percent perfume concentrates. This makes for a light scent that doesn't linger as long as the more intense versions. It was originally intended to be a refreshing body splash to help people wake up in the morning.

- *Eau de cologne* is sometimes used interchangeably with the term eau de toilette. However, the concoction began as the name of a light, fresh fragrance mixed with citrus oils and was made popular by Napoleon. Some perfumers today have a version of this called *eau fraiche.*[1]

The higher the concentrate of perfume, the higher the price. Subsequently, however, the higher the price—typically—the more staying power the scent has. But if you have dry skin,

When it comes to fragrance, author and speaker
Denise Hildreth (Savannah from Savannah series) and
wife of Christian recording artist Jonathan Pierce, says,
"I have two—one for the summer and one for the
winter. Summer is Vera Wang by Vera Wang because it
is more floral. Winter is Burberry by Burberry because it
is more musky. But Jonathan went and messed me up
when he bought me a third for Christmas, Calvin Klein's
Euphoria. So I have no idea what I'm going to do now."

your time may be lessened no matter what. Moisture in the
skin helps to hold on to the fragrance. Another good reason
to layer.

It's not unusual for women to have signature fragrances
that change with the season. Lighter fragrances for spring
and summer, heavier for fall and winter. It's also common
for women to have an "everyday" scent versus the "evening
out" or "special occasion" scents. Personally, when I'm
home, I use a variety of body lotions and body sprays in
citrus, with my special-occasion choice being more oriental
or floral. Whatever you choose, just make sure you don't
drown yourself in the stuff. Others will be offended, not
pleased, and causing offense is not the purpose of wearing fragrance. (Note: in some cases, as when working in
closed settings, those around you may be allergic to scent.
Be sensitive to their needs in this, as any true lady of the
Lord would.)

The Body Beautiful—Spiritual

Then Mary took about a pint of pure nard, an expensive
perfume; she poured it on Jesus' feet and wiped his feet

with her hair. And the house was filled with the fragrance of the perfume.

John 12:3

It had been a long journey. One hundred and twenty years of preparation as neighbors and family and friends no doubt laughed and mocked the boat builder. "Rain?" they scoffed. "A flood?"

Ark completed, Noah and his small family—a wife, three sons, and three daughters-in-law—climbed aboard with pairs of animals. Four human couples, no telling how many of the other kind. And then the rain came, and the whole earth was flooded. Noah and his family most likely heard the cries of the people and the animals not chosen as, one by one, they drowned. They felt the ark as it began to float and then rock back and forth under the influence of the strong waves.

The rain stopped. The floodwaters remained. For days . . . weeks . . . months . . . over a year, the tiny family and the animals waited inside. Waited and waited. Was there tension? Arguments over who would muck the stalls? Were children born, human or other? It couldn't all have been playing shuffleboard on the Ledo deck.

Finally the land was completely dry. God said, "Come out," and they did. Noah, his wife, his sons, and his sons' wives. Behind them, the animals. Two by two. Maybe an occasional "three-sie."

What did Noah do next? Throw a welcome-home party? No. Call his Realtor in hopes that some beachfront property had become available for purchase? No. He built an altar to the Lord and sacrificed a burnt offering of *clean* (and therefore acceptable and pleasing) animals on it.

The Lord smelled the pleasing aroma . . .

In the books of Exodus, Leviticus, and Numbers, we read of the provisions God gave for sacrifice, something he called a "pleasing aroma," and of various sacrifices that were made to him. Some were voluntary acts of worship and thanksgiving. Others were mandatory and for the atonement of sin. Either way, when the sacrifice was made, the aroma would reach the nostrils of Jehovah and was pleasing to him.

Thousands of years would pass and countless sacrifices would be made until God himself came to earth in the form of a baby boy, born to a poor Jewish *tekton* (Greek, often translated "carpenter") named Joseph and his wife, Mary, a young Jewish girl.

He would grow up and follow in his earthly father's footsteps, taking on the same trade. He would care for his mother and sisters and brothers in the absence of Joseph. Then, at the age of about thirty, he would leave it all behind and come to the fullness of himself as Messiah. For three and a half years he would walk the Galilean and Judean countryside, preaching the love of the Father. He would heal those who were sick and raise to life those who had died.

One of the deceased was his friend Lazarus. Lazarus and his two sisters, Mary and Martha, were all beloved of Jesus. The Gospel of John is very specific about his affection for the siblings. "Jesus loved Martha and her sister and Lazarus" (John 11:5). When Jesus received word that Lazarus was sick, however, he waited two more days before returning to Judea, where Lazarus lived, specifically in the village of Bethany.

When Jesus arrived, he was immediately met by Martha, who—in her characteristic way—spouted, "Lord, if you had been here, my brother would not have died."

After a bit of conversation, Jesus sent Martha to get Mary, who had sat at his feet previously, listening to his words and teachings while Martha slaved like a madwoman in the kitchen. (See Luke 10.) Mary came and, *falling at his feet*, said, "Lord, if you had been here, my brother would not have died."

Same words as her sister, different position.

Sitting at the feet of Jesus during good times enables us to fall at his feet during the bad times.

Mary began to weep, the kind of crying that is more of a wail than mere tears streaming down your cheeks. The kind that comes from the very pit of yourself when you feel that there is nothing left to live for, no understanding of life at all.

Jesus, so moved by her emotion, asked to be taken to where Lazarus's body was. When he came to the tomb, he said, "Lazarus, come out!"

And Lazarus did.

No doubt there was much to celebrate. No doubt Martha learned about worshiping at the feet of Jesus. No doubt Mary fell more deeply in love with her Creator than she could have ever imagined.

Some time later—six days before his last Passover on earth—Jesus was at the home of the siblings. Martha served a dinner prepared in Jesus' honor while Lazarus reclined at the table with the One who had breathed life into him as an

> You are a garden locked up, my sister, my bride; you are a spring enclosed, a sealed fountain. Your plants are an orchard of pomegranates with choice fruits, with henna and nard, nard and saffron, calamus and cinnamon, with every kind of incense tree, with myrrh and aloes and all the finest spices.
>
> Song of Songs 4:12–14

embryo and then spoke it into him from outside a cave. Oh, there must have been a houseful of joy and celebration that evening.

Then, in a touching move that has placed her in the remembrance of millions, Mary came in with a pint of pure nard, which is an expensive (and therefore a sacrifice for her) perfume with an intense, warm, and musky fragrance. Kneeling, she poured it on Jesus' feet, then unbound her hair and began to wipe.

When she was rebuked for her actions, Jesus hushed them, telling them that what she had done would prepare him for his death. His voluntary sacrifice for the forgiveness of our sins.

John writes, "And the house was filled with the fragrance of the perfume" (John 12:2).

How sweet it must have smelled. How pleasing to the Lord.

But was it the perfume from the nard . . . or from Mary's act of worship and sacrifice?

When you worship, is it pleasing to the Lord? Is it pure? Are you quick to fall at his feet in times of gaiety and joy as well as in times of distress? Are you happy just to listen to his words, to what he has to say about your life? Are you willing to trust him, even in the face of death? Would you pour out of your heart, as Mary poured out of the alabaster box holding the nard? Or do you keep things so tightly shut

Allison M. Wilson, a mom from Palm Bay, Florida, says, "I wear Henri Bendel—Vanilla Flower. I like the lightness of the scent. I can wear it all day and not get tired of it. It's also light enough for me to wear without bothering people near me with overpowering vapors."

in that you think he can't see them? Would you be willing to forsake what anyone else might think and lay your life on the altar as he did? To call yourself his beloved? To have him call you the same?

Questions for Personal Reflection or Group Study

1. Do you have a favorite perfume? What is it?
2. Do you use a different scent for "around the house" versus "outside of the house"?
3. Think about the perfume you wore as a teenager. How is it different from the fragrance you wear today?
4. Use the questions in the last paragraph of "The Body Beautiful—Spiritual" as a guide for group discussion or personal journaling.
5. Read these words out loud: "For we are to God the aroma of Christ among those who are being saved and those who are perishing" (2 Cor. 2:15). What do those words mean to you?

Here's a Valuable Tip

Perfume should be applied to the "pulse spots" of your body: wrists, throat (feel for the heartbeat), temples, and even behind the knees. Your body heat and the beating of your heart will help it to do what it was created to do. If it comes in a bottle that requires you to apply it with your finger, be sure your hands are clean. Between applications, keep the bottle tightly sealed and away from hot places or sunlight.

14

FASHION

I delight greatly in the LORD;
   my soul rejoices in my God.
For he has clothed me with garments of salvation
   and arrayed me in a robe of righteousness,
as a bridegroom adorns his head like a priest,
   and as a bride adorns herself with her jewels.

Isaiah 61:10

I love clothes. I love shopping for them, I love trying them on (except when I've put on a few pounds here and there), and I love wearing them (aren't you glad?). The only time I get aggravated with clothes is when:

A. I need a special outfit for a special event and can't find anything (and I do mean anything) at the shopping centers, vast as they may be in my area.
B. I've gained those notorious few pounds, and I now need to lose five to ten pounds in thirty seconds—so I can wear the killer outfit to the event.
C. My closet seems suddenly filled to the brim with absolutely nothing I want to wear. These are the times

Ramona Richards, an editor from Nashville, Tennessee, says, "My word, at age forty-eight I've become 'femmy'; I've fallen in love with cute shoes and purses. After decades of carrying the same oversized black leather purse everywhere and wearing the same sensible shoes, I guess I'm in midlife adolescence."

you'll hear me cry out, "I have nothing to wear! Nothing, I tell you! Nothing!"

This, of course, results in a shopping trip.

Now, speaking of shopping, I also love finding great bargains on good clothes. There's such a markup, you know. And, I enjoy putting together outfits for the different areas of my life. I learned a long time ago that even a sweat suit can look sharp when worn correctly (we'll talk more about that later).

The Body Beautiful—Physical

I clothed you with an embroidered dress and put leather sandals on you. I dressed you in fine linen and covered you with costly garments.

Ezekiel 16:10

Here's what I've discovered. Women either love clothes or they hate them. Or, at least they think they do. The truth of the matter is, they either love the way they look in them or they hate the way they look in them. Clothes can make all the difference in a woman's day. A day could be headed south faster than Rear Admiral Richard E. Byrd flying toward Antarctica; but then put on a sharp outfit—one that fits well and looks good—and the whole day suddenly looks brighter.

You've no doubt heard the old saying "You are what you eat." If that's true, is it not equally true that we are what we wear? Think about it. Don't the majority of us try to express something about our personalities through what we call "fashion"?

We call them "fashion statements," and they are exactly that: a statement. What we wear is really about image and lifestyle.

> Clothes make the man. Naked people have little or no influence on society.
>
> Mark Twain

Whenever I go shopping for clothes—and especially when I go with a friend—I find that there are two questions pulsating through my mind as I pull hangers draped with new finds from racks and stands.

1. How will I look to others?
2. How will I—personally—feel in it, both literally and figuratively?

How Will I Look to Others?

Be honest. Aren't others who we really choose our clothes for? Recently, after a weight loss, I found myself happier slipping into a pair of jeans than I'd been in a long time. My husband was pretty giddy too; he loves the way I look in jeans. On the plus side, I like wearing jeans—they're comfy—so jeans became a serious focal point of my wardrobe. More because of my husband's thrill than my comfort, however.

Most of us—whether we're dressing for the office or for church or for a special dinner or occasion out—think, *What will others say I look like in this?* At no time is this truer than at high school or college reunions. We will spend days shopping for that perfect outfit. Price becomes no object. We'll give up our daily Starbucks for a month if we have to in order to have extra greenbacks. And then we'll make a big mistake: we'll purchase a size smaller than we should in hopes that we really will exercise a bit more and eat a bit less so we can squeeze into it.

And why? Because *others* will see us and will "judge" how we look.

Our workplaces can become fashion halls as well. Businesswomen can spot a name-brand suit from six cubicles away or all the way down a mile-long conference table. Fact is, other businesswomen know this, so they dress appropriately. That name brand screams "success." In the business world, success is everything. Otherwise, what's the point?

> Ever wonder why you're a size 8 but can't manage to squeeze into your mother's vintage size 10 skirt? That's because a size 10 from 1942 is equivalent to a size 2 today.
> Marie Claire, jaehakim.com/articles/misc/features/sizes.htm

Even soccer fields and ballet halls can become fashion runways. There are websites dedicated to soccer moms and their sense of style. I mean, how cool is that? (And who would have ever believed it could be so?)

Finally, what is exercise class but a way to sweat in style? When my walking buddy and I first began walking together in order to shed that unwanted and unwelcome extra poundage that had attacked from the rear (and from the waist down), we were happy to pull on sloppy sweats and an over-sized man's oxford shirt worn over a large tee. But when the walking produced results, we suddenly found ourselves shopping for what we insisted was appropriate sportswear.

From that day on, we walked in style.

Because we actually care what others think—and you're lying if you say you don't—you'll want to make certain you use your clothes to draw attention to your best features and away from your not-so-best. This is accomplished with lines, colors, and fabrics. You'll also want to remember your age. What looks good on a twenty-one-year-old won't look the same on a fifty-one-year-old. Does that mean that a twenty-one-year-old has one over on the fifty-one-year-old? No way. While it's true that the older we get the more our unflattering features tend to rise up (or, fall down) and scream, "Look at me!" it doesn't mean that we have to become fashion victims or the cause for jokes.

How Will I—Personally—Feel in It?

Some fabrics I won't even bother to try on, and for good reason; they don't "fit" right. Sure, I would have worn them in my twenties, but not now. When it comes to fashion sense, you have to use common sense in order for it to work.

> Clothes should glide, drape, over the body, never hug or require pulling or tugging to keep them in place.
> Gale Hayman,
> *How Do I Look?*

In her book *How Do I Look?* Gale Hayman—the cofounder of Giorgio, Beverly Hills—states, "Most fashion-savvy clients never squeezed themselves into clothes but always bought them one size bigger to make them look slimmer."[1] For some reason, women have erroneously believed that the tighter the fit, the thinner they look.

I learned my lesson a long time ago.

It was a perfect spring afternoon; my daughters and I were playing in the front yard of our home. My best friend's car pulled up, and she waved hello as she stepped out of the car and strolled toward us.

"Have you lost weight?" I asked, noting immediately that my already-thin friend looked even slimmer than usual.

"Oh no," she said, tugging at the waistband. "I'm wearing my sister's jeans, and she's a size larger than me." Then she chuckled a bit. "I know one thing, they feel a lot better than my tight jeans."

"Well," I said, "feel good or not, they make you look thinner."

Can you think of anything more miserable than spending all day wearing an outfit that is ill fitting, whether too tight, too loose, too short, or too long? By the end of the day you're not sure if you've worn your clothes or if they've worn you.

When trying on clothes, pay special attention to what I call the Four Ss.

Shoulders. Look at the lines. They shouldn't drape beyond your shoulder blades. Clean lines are what you want.

Sleeves. If you are wearing long sleeves, make certain the sleeves meet the wrists.

Seams. How do the seams lie against the body? Let's say you're wearing a skirt with side seams. Look closely; where are those seams? They should run along the sides of your legs and not be catawampus.

Skirt/slacks hems. Make certain hems are where they need to be. If you are horizontally challenged (aka, short), you will most likely have to have the hems of your skirts, dresses, or slacks altered. Same goes if you are horizontally blessed (aka, tall).

You can save yourself a lot of misery by first reminding yourself that size does not matter. Then, educate yourself.

All designers cut fabric differently, so one designer's size 6 is another designer's size 8. To make it all a bit more complicated, a single designer can cut two styles of the same type of clothing in a different way, thereby changing the size. Said simply, two pair of slacks in size 10 won't necessarily both fit you. So take a moment and try them on. Don't stress over the size. The question to answer is "How do I feel in it?" not "What size is inked into the label?"

Fashion Rules

Rule #1. Your wardrobe is divided into three "who you are" sections.

1. **Who you are at home.** This is what you wear around the house. Jeans. Shorts. Exercise clothes. Casual dresses. Your choice. Just make them comfortable.
2. **Who you are away from home.** This is what you wear to the office, to the soccer field, to the grocery store, to church, and everywhere in between.
3. **Who you are after dark.** Whether you're attending a special dinner or going to the theater and/or how you dress in the privacy of your boudoir. (P.S. Mother and I have always "dressed for bed" whether married or single, but that's our choice. That's who we are.) Whether you choose sweats for bed or elegant lingerie, this is "who you are after dark."

Rule #2. Learn to read labels, everything from the fabrics to fabric care. Especially the Dry Clean Only label. Many a nice outfit has been trashed after being washed when it should never have seen a drop of water.

Rule #3. Keep the truly necessary items—an iron, lint

> When it comes to fashion, author and speaker Rose Sweet (*Dear God, Send Me a Soul Mate*) sticks to fashion, not fads. "I have spent thousands of dollars over the years on fads that fade. No more!" Her favorite designer? "St. John Knits are classic, with timeless lines and quality that fits all shapes and rarely goes out of style. For less expensive/more casual I love Jones of New York. Very classy."

brush, sweater comb, plastic bags—in your closet (or fairly close).

Rule #4. Pay attention to your underwear! Before you walk out the door, make sure your panty lines aren't showing and your bra straps are in place. (I am notorious for this. Bra straps and I just don't get along for some reason, so I try to pay special attention to them.) Remember to wear slips to keep sheer fabrics from showing all the possibilities and to keep outer fabrics sleek and smooth.

Rule #5. Go beyond this year's fad. Think *fashion*. Purchase clothes with *style*.

Rule #6. When you shop, go armed with more than a credit card or your checkbook. Take your common sense along too. Before you purchase, know for certain that you'll wear the clothes and that the color is right for you.

The Body Beautiful—Spiritual

> Be dressed ready for service and keep your lamps burning, like men waiting for their master to return from a wedding banquet, so that when he comes and knocks they can immediately open the door for him.
>
> Luke 12:35–36

Have you ever thought that you'd like to have your own personal shopper? Let's pretend, shall we? Okay, you're a hotshot executive who barely has time to breathe, much less shop. However, you've been invited to the Party of the Year. A look into your closet and . . . my goodness . . . not a thing to wear! (Which is hardly true, but rather a line women like to use when they don't like the way they look in many of their clothes or they haven't shopped in a while.) You could wear the little black beaded thing, but you wore that to the last social function. You could wear the sharp red dress, but someone told you they saw So-and-So wearing one just like it at the big company dinner you missed because you were in Europe hobnobbing with the British executive snobs. Oh, dear. What to do?

Never fear! A quick call to your personal shopper will have this dilemma all taken care of. You tell her that you need a dress to die for, shoes to match, a purse that kills, and something really fabulous to wear on your head. A hat or a tiara; you're not overly picky, for crying out loud.

Now that we've had a little fun with that scenario, let me present another one. You're a child of the King. A member of royalty. It's not enough to wear your everyday or even your workout clothes. You want to dress like someone who knows she's going to spend eternity walking on streets of gold.

Now allow me to be your personal shopper. A quick dash into Isaiah's House of Style, and we find this in the storefront window:

> The Spirit of the Sovereign LORD is on me,
>> because the LORD has anointed me
>> to preach good news to the poor.
> He has sent me to bind up the brokenhearted,
>> to proclaim freedom for the captives
>> and release from darkness for the prisoners,

to proclaim the year of the LORD's favor
    and the day of vengeance of our God,
to comfort all who mourn,
    and provide for those who grieve in Zion—
to bestow on them a crown of beauty
    instead of ashes,
the oil of gladness
    instead of mourning,
and a *garment of praise*
    instead of a spirit of despair.
They will be called oaks of righteousness,
    a planting of the LORD
    for the display of his splendor.

Isaiah 61:1–3, emphasis mine

The word used for *garment* in Isaiah is the Hebrew *ma`ateh*, from which we get the word *mantle*. A mantle is more than something you wear; it is something you wrap around your body.

I love to get up early in the morning, make a pot of coffee, and then—steaming cup in hand—step out onto the screened patio of our home. During the winter months I wrap a throw—a big thick one—around me. I am literally engulfed in it. I am warm and protected against the elements, and as far as I'm concerned, very little can compare with these moments because these are the precious minutes I spend with the Lord before the rest of the world rises and interrupts our time.

The garment of praise is much like this. It is a mantle that wraps around the whole person. The praise itself seems to swirl and dance and rise up to heaven. One becomes engulfed, or protected by it.

How does one put on the garment of praise? Do you slip it over your arms or step into it? Well, of course that's a facetious question. Or, is it? Personally, I slip it over my arms by raising them high (whether literally or figuratively) and then by beginning my long list of thank-yous to my heavenly Father, the giver of all good things. Not one single "And please, Lord, if it's in your will, do thus and such for me." No. This is a time for PRAISE!

Thank you! Thank you! Thank you!

Moses wrote (actually he sang!): "The LORD is my strength and my song; he has become my salvation. He is my God, and I will *praise him*, my father's God, and I will exalt him" (Exod. 15:2, emphasis mine).

David wrote (and sang and wrote and sang) the words *praise him* in so many of his psalms—or songs—of love and devotion, but also in his words of anguish and pain. "Let the righteous rejoice in the LORD and take refuge in him; let all the upright in heart *praise him*!" (Ps. 64:10, emphasis mine). "*Praise* be to the LORD, for he has heard my cry for mercy" (Ps. 28:6, emphasis mine).

David, like you and me, had so much to be grateful for, but he, like you and me, had much to mourn. In his lifetime he gained and lost much. He truly experienced life at its best and worst. And yet, he *praised* the Lord and was known as a man who sought after the heart of God (1 Sam. 13:14; Acts 13:22).

God inhabits or is enthroned on the praises of his people, according to Psalm 22:3. When we praise, he comes and wraps himself around us like a mantle. Or, like a garment of praise!

Back to shopping with your personal shopper. Next stop: Ephesians by Paul. Here we'll pick up a little something for your feet. "Stand firm then . . . with your *feet fitted* with the readiness that comes from the gospel of peace" (Eph. 6:14–15, emphasis mine).

While we'll talk more about feet later, let me just throw this in for your consideration: ever worn ill-fitting shoes? A year and a half ago, while in Israel, one of my fellow journalists wore shoes that were not meant for a lot of walking. We'd been driven everywhere by our trusty little driver (who looked remarkably like Danny DeVito with a long ponytail). But on this particular day it was Shabbat, and, as our driver was an observant Jew, our feet became our transportation for the day.

Now, when I say we "climbed Mt. Zion," I mean it. Nearing the end of the day, my fellow journalist began to limp. In fact, her heels were literally bleeding. It was just awful, and, naturally, every one of us could empathize. At one time or another we've worn shoes that didn't fit right . . . or pinched . . . or were painful to the balls of the feet. A cab was hailed, and the injured tourist was whisked away to our hotel for a good foot soaking.

Unlike those ill-fitting shoes, the gospel of peace fits perfectly. It is so comfortable, in fact, one can "run the race" with ne'er a "foot" problem to whine about.

Last stop: another mad dash back to Isaiah's House of Style. The "garment of praise" and the "shoes of peace" demand the perfect accessories, and I know just where to get them. Department 61:10 displays the following: "I will sing for joy in God, explode in praise from deep in my soul! He dressed me up in a suit of salvation, he outfitted me in a robe of righteousness, as a bridegroom who puts on a tuxedo and a bride a *jeweled tiara*" (Message, emphasis mine).

I love the way this verse has been translated. "I . . . explode in praise from deep in my soul! He dressed me up in a suit of salvation . . . a robe of righteousness. . . ."

Are you grasping this? Stand before the mirror, that famous three-sided mirror every good shopping experience needs, and gaze upon the beauty of a Christian dressed in praise and peace, salvation and righteousness. Darling, you look marvelous!

But before we just leave you standing there gazing at your own beauty, allow me—your personal shopper—to whisper something in your ear. "He dressed me up in a suit of salvation, he outfitted me in a robe of righteousness, as a bridegroom who puts on a tuxedo and a bride a jeweled tiara."

That function you (and I) have been invited to is the wedding of the Lamb, my friend.

> Then I heard what sounded like a great multitude, like the roar of rushing waters and like loud peals of thunder, shouting: "Hallelujah! For our Lord God almighty reigns. Let us rejoice and be glad and give him glory! For the wedding of the Lamb has come, and his bride has made herself ready. Fine linen, bright and clean, was given her to wear." [Fine linen stands for the righteous acts of the saints.] Then the angel said to me, "Write: 'Blessed are those who are invited to the wedding supper of the Lamb!'" And he added, "These are the true words of God."
>
> Revelation 15:6–9

Fine linen is not often mentioned in the Bible, but when it is . . . look out! It's impressively important.

Do you remember the story of the Old Testament Joseph? Sold into slavery by his brothers, worked in the home of the Egyptian Potiphar, was falsely accused of attempted rape by Potiphar's wife, served time in prison but was then elevated to a high position within the Egyptian government. When this happened, the Word tells us, "Then Pharaoh took his signet ring from his finger and put it on Joseph's finger.

He dressed him in robes of *fine linen* and put a gold chain around his neck" (Gen. 41:42, emphasis mine).

Fine linen was also draped on Mordecai, the uncle of the Old Testament Esther, when the Jewish people had been saved from the death sentence proposed by the scheming Haman. (Read the book of Esther. It'll only take a few minutes.) The Bible tells us that the entire city of Susa rejoiced and shouted and that there was celebration filled with gladness, joy, and honor (see Esther 8:15–17).

The curtains of the tabernacle were made of fine linen, and the vestments of the priests were also made of fine linen, as were their turbans and headbands. "Make tunics, sashes and headbands for Aaron's sons, *to give them dignity and honor*" (Exod. 28:40, emphasis mine).

Finally, the Great High Priest, Jesus our Bridegroom, was wrapped in fine linen when he was laid within the tomb from which he would rise three days later.

> Joseph of Arimathea, a prominent member of the Council, who was himself waiting for the kingdom of God, went boldly to Pilate and asked for Jesus' body. . . . Joseph bought some linen cloth, took down the body, wrapped it in the linen, and placed it in a tomb cut out of rock. Then he rolled a stone against the entrance of the tomb.
>
> Mark 15:43, 46

Is it any wonder then that the bride of Christ will be dressed in fine linen, which represents her righteous acts, as it has also been associated with honor, gladness, joy, prominence, and, above all, that which wrapped itself around the body of Christ as the whole world waited for the Son of God's return?

Much as we wait today.

Questions for Personal Reflection or Group Study

1. If someone looked into your closet, what would they surmise about your fashion sense?
2. When folks look at you, what do you think they surmise about your spiritual fashion sense?

Diane Floate, a stay-at-home mom and substitute teacher from Huntsville, Alabama, says, "Oh, girlfriend, let me tell you about my fashion makeover! Several months ago, I decided I was tired of wearing the same ole, same ole. I decided to go out and purchase some new clothing. I didn't do it all at once. I just started putting together some of the old and some of the new and some in between and voila!—Di's new look! I can't tell you how many comments and compliments I have received. My clothing style consists of putting together an outfit of something casual such as a 100-percent cotton skirt with a little something 'fancy' or dressy to be precise, a ruffled, gathered, and kinda silky blouse with a short denim jacket thrown on top for 'flava.' Oh, I almost forgot my cowboy boots complete the ensemble. Well, the compliments have poured in; even teen girls from church are coming up and telling me that they have decided when they grow up they want to be Mrs. Floate. I have to admit it does make you feel kinda warm and toasty inside. Oh, one of the best things about the new 'look'—it hides all the little flaws and not-so-little flaws we all get as we grow a little older."

3. Take a look at the following words:
   a. Peace
   b. Praise
   c. Salvation
   d. Righteousness
   Write out what you think these words mean.
4. Now look at these same words with their Hebrew/Greek meanings.[2] How were your definitions similar? How were they different?

   Peace (Greek: *eirene*; pronounced: *i-ray'-nay*) of Christianity: the tranquil state of a soul assured of its salvation through Christ, and so fearing nothing from God and being content with its earthly lot, of whatsoever sort that is

   Praise (Hebrew: *tehillah*; pronounced: *teh-hil-law'*): praise, song, or hymn of praise, adoration, thanksgiving (to God)

   Salvation (Hebrew: *yesha'*; pronounced: *yeh'-shah*): deliverance, salvation, rescue, safety, welfare, prosperity, victory

   Righteousness (Greek: *dikaiosune*; pronounced: *dik-ah-yos-oo'-nay*): the doctrine concerning the way in which man may attain a state approved of God; integrity, virtue, purity of life, rightness, correctness of thinking, feeling, and acting

Here's a Valuable Tip

In the movie *Steel Magnolias*, Clairee Belcher (played by Olympia Dukakis) declares, "The only thing that separates us from the animals is our ability to accessorize." When it comes to fashion, don't stop with the obvious. Throw a silver chain belt on a pair of plain slacks, and you've got pizzazz. Add a brooch to a jacket and make it sharp. Add drop-pearl earrings and a necklace set to that little black dress, and you've got stunning. A shimmery top and some pointy dress shoes added to a pair of jeans, and you've got style!

Accessorize . . . and set yourself apart.

15

STAYING FIT
FOR THE JOURNEY

Do you not know that in a race all the runners run, but only
one gets the prize? Run in such a way as to get the prize.

1 Corinthians 9:24

Years ago I worked as a behavioral health educator. What
that means is this: I taught people how to have healthy, active lifestyles based on their eating and exercise habits. Out
of all the jobs I've ever had, this one was by far my favorite
and the most fun! (With the exception of writing and speaking, of course.) It was exciting to see people—previously
unhealthy, lethargic, and tied to their next meal—become
healthy, energized, and educated on eating right.

Initially, as patients came to the institute, I would help
them assess their exercise needs. Part of this included noting their current fitness habits.

I'll never forget the afternoon I sat in my office with a new
patient. She had meticulously listed every bite of food she'd
eaten the previous week in one column and her exercise

> Debby Henry, a full-time wife and mom and part-time freelance writer from Winter Springs, Florida, says, "I'm always doing something—usually running more than anything—but I also taught kickboxing at the Y at one point, and my latest love is Tai Kwon Do. I view exercise as a way of staying emotionally fit just as much as physically fit."

patterns for the week in another. Imagine my expression when, on her very first day, she'd listed "feeding my cats" as her exercise regimen.

I pressed my lips together to keep from laughing, then excused myself and stepped into the hallway, closing the office door behind me. I walked around the corner and came face-to-face with the institute's chief physician. "What's the matter?" he asked me, sensing my "how am I going to address this?" turmoil.

I showed him the entry.

"What kind of cats does she have?" he asked. "Tigers?"

Clearly, this was a patient who knew very little about living the active lifestyle, and my work was cut out for me!

The Body Beautiful—Physical

Therefore, since we are surrounded by such a great cloud of witnesses, let us throw off everything that hinders and the sin that so easily entangles, and let us run with perseverance the race marked out for us.

Hebrews 12:1

I probably don't have to tell you the benefits of exercise. Books have been written about it. TV shows have been dedicated to it. Talk radio has laid it all out for us. But, for the one or two of you out there who have been living under a rock and haven't heard, here are but a few paybacks of a lifestyle of regular exercise:

1. Exercise increases your chance of weight loss.
2. Exercise decreases your chance of heart disease.
3. Exercise decreases your chance of stroke.
4. Exercise increases stress management.
5. Exercise slows the aging process.
6. Exercise increases self-esteem and confidence.
7. Exercise helps you sleep.
8. Exercise steps up your immune system.
9. Exercise reduces the chance of your contracting various cancers.
10. Exercise improves your overall quality of life.

There's another benefit. A few years ago, while sitting at a café snacking on chocolate cake and coffee, a good friend and I were bemoaning our weight gain. Struck by a sudden case of "the guilts," we both vowed to begin watching our caloric intake (like I needed to be told this!) and then set a walking program we could follow together.

A few days later, clad in sweats and walking shoes, we began our new regimen. We walked a mile, prayed we'd be able to make it back to her house, and then the next day repeated the torture. But, within a couple of weeks, we had moved up to two miles . . . then three. At one time, we were doing four miles (until our schedules went completely crazy). Eventually we settled on two to three miles a day, four to five days a week. When, again, our schedules went nuts and we were unable to meet, we continued our walking, but separately.

Our greatest benefit? No, not the weight loss (though that has been wonderful!). No, not the closeness we've come to feel as our friendship has deepened. Our greatest benefit has been the times we have prayed together, lifting each other up before the throne of grace and mercy as we pound the pavement.

One of the easiest things to do when it comes to exercise is to *say* you're going to do it. One of the most difficult is to stick with it. Here are a few tips that will help you start and stick with an exercise program:

1. Find a partner. Keep each other accountable.
2. Whatever exercise you pick, make it something you love to do. If you are not a runner, don't choose jogging. If you are afraid of water, I'd suggest you not choose swimming (which, by the way, is an excellent form of exercise and one I do with my granddaughter all spring and summer long).
3. Pick the right time of day. If you are a runner or walker, like I am, don't wait until the heat of the day. Instead, choose mornings or evenings. If you live in a cold climate, be conscious of your clothing.
4. Start off slow. This isn't the Olympics, and you're not representing the United States. This is for you. Take your time . . . enjoy . . .
5. Remember, a little soreness can be expected . . . but you should not be in agony. If you want an easy way to convince yourself to stop exercising, injury would be at the top of the list.

Finally, if you have not been active in a while, are elderly, pregnant, or have certain physical disabilities, be sure to speak to your physician before beginning any type of program, including those you might feel are "easy." Together

When it comes to exercise, author, speaker, and president of CLASS Marita Littauer (*Wired That Way*) says, "My favorite form of exercise is rollerblading. It's perfect for me because I can do it by myself, whenever it fits into my schedule. I don't have to pay gym fees or endure the smell of the sweat. Whether I rollerblade for thirty minutes or three hours, it gives me a good workout while enjoying nature. There is a twenty-three-mile trail along the Rio Grande in Albuquerque that is perfect for biking and blading. Whenever I blade along the trail, I am encouraged that there is hope for humanity as it is filled (on weekends) with families biking, walking the dog, or participating in other normal activities. Plus roller blades are easier to pack for travel than a bicycle (my husband's exercise of choice)."

you should be able to design a program that is right for you.

The Body Beautiful—Spiritual

For bodily discipline is only of little profit, but godliness is profitable for all things, since it holds promise for the present life and also for the life to come.

1 Timothy 4:8 NASB

I've heard this verse misquoted many times. "The Bible says you shouldn't exercise," someone told me, citing the above Scripture. Ah, no. Paul was expressing the difference in the physical body's ability to further the kingdom versus what's on the inside being fit enough to do the same. He was also speaking to a people who put a lot of stock in physical fitness. Paul is not saying physical discipline is wrong but instead that godliness holds an even greater promise.

So, then, what is this godliness we should be striving toward as diligently as we push ourselves toward physical "perfection"?

I spent a lot of time one weekend studying the word *godliness*. And, as you might have guessed, I spent a lot of time being spiritually challenged on the principles of godly behavior. Everything that could go wrong did go wrong, and in the absolute worst way. At one point I threw up my arms and cried out, "Why did you have to choose me for this life? Why couldn't you just leave me alone . . . let me be?"

Thank the good Lord, he knew I didn't mean a word of it! But was that godly behavior? Not for a moment. So, I persisted in study, finally resting on the words of Peter in 1 Peter, beginning at 1:13 and continuing until 5:11. The NIV study notes state that these verses are "imperatives" for holy living. For sure, holiness is godliness because God is holy (Ps. 99:9).

The content of these verses is difficult. The words are many. But I encourage you to sit down with pad and pen and write down the instructions Peter gave for holy living. *A holy life.* As you do, note 1 Peter 3:15, which reads: "But in your hearts set apart Christ as Lord."

This is the absolute first step to living a godly life. If Christ is not Lord, there is no point . . . there is no hope . . . there is no way!

Also notice that many of the imperatives given by Peter are followed with "because" or "so that." In other words, cause and effect. Just as physical exercise has results and benefits, so too does the spiritual "exercise" of holy living. For example, 1 Peter 2:2: "Like newborn babies, crave pure spiritual milk, *so that* by it you may grow up in your salvation." And 1 Peter 4:8: "Above all, love each other deeply, *because* love covers over a multitude of sins" (emphasis mine).

As you pore over the verses of godly living, you may think, "I could never accomplish all this! I could never be this . . . this . . . *godly!*"

This would be like me looking at a photo of fitness guru Cory Everson (Get it? *Everson?*) and saying, "I could never look like that! No matter how many miles I walked or crunches I groaned through."

No. I may never reach physical perfection in this lifetime (but I've got some pretty firm hopes for heaven, let me tell you!), but it won't keep me from doing whatever I need to do to stay as toned as possible.

Spiritual exercise—this workout toward becoming godly—requires a one-two punch.

Punch Number One. When I wanted to become physically fit (or, in my case, less unfit), I grabbed a walking/accountability partner. We should do the same in our quest to be spiritually fit. Actually, we should grab two—the first being the Holy Spirit. Without him, we won't make it past this first imperative. With him we can do all things (Phil. 4:13).

Punch Number Two. We should have a prayer/accountability partner, making sure this is someone who is spiritually on the same level as we are and someone who wants to live a godly life as much as we do. Obviously, we should feel secure that this is someone trustworthy, never forgetting that we are there for each other, not just that "she is there for me." Our trustworthiness must also be as firm as we want our legs to be.

Charlene Elder, an administrative assistant from Woodstock, Georgia, says, "To stay healthy and active, you should make exercise an important part of your life. I'm nearly fifty-eight years old, and I've used everything from the exercise ball, to rebounding (which is great), to treadmill walking, to Tae Bo, to using Core Secrets tapes, and weights to keep in shape."

Questions for Personal Reflection or Group Study

1. How physically fit are you?
2. What kind of physical exercise do you enjoy? How often do you participate in this?
3. Do you have an accountability partner for your physical fitness goals? Why or why not?
4. How spiritually fit are you? Do you have an accountability partner for your spiritual fitness goals? Why or why not?
5. Read 1 Peter. List all the imperatives you find within the verses.
6. In a separate list, note those Scriptures that give a "result."
7. When you look at the first list, how "godly" are you? Where are your strongest areas? Your weakest? What goals can you set to become more spiritually strong?

Here's a Valuable Tip

Sometimes I hear women say that they are physically active in their jobs and that this should be enough. Mothers chasing after toddlers. Salesclerks running around for customers. Teachers standing on their feet all day. Nurses and doctors going up and down the hospital corridors. The list goes on and on.

But whatever you do daily is what your body will adapt to. And, it's "old hat."

Exercise should be something away from the drudgery of your job. (Or, the day-to-day-ness of your job, if your job is not drudgery at all.) Exercise should be something that allows you to free your mind from all that is weighty in life. Something that allows you to breathe and breathe big.

When it comes to exercise, it's easy to say, "I'll start tomorrow." Or, even, "I'll do it tomorrow."

But, it's just as easy to say, "I'll do it right now."

So go on. Get out there. Be fit for the journey!

A FINAL WORD
ABOUT THE BODY BEAUTIFUL

What you have read began as a series of articles for Cross walk.com. In twelve installments I gave women across the world a look at taking care of their physical bodies and how this relates to their spiritual bodies.

I'll be honest with you. I didn't want to write the articles. I felt like people would call me vain. Ungodly. Destined for the opposite of the pearly gates. But, I kept talking to my editor about it, and she kept saying, "Do it, Eva! Today's Christian woman battles this issue. Do it!"

So I did it. I wrote the articles. The number of emails I have received has been overwhelming. Women thanking me profusely. Telling me they'd been brought to a deeper understanding of taking care of themselves *spiritually*.

I did receive two negative emails. Out of all of the good ones, just two. Both assumed I am a woman of "means" with money to burn. Let me assure you I am not. I have found that taking care of myself doesn't cost nearly as much as it rewards, and "dime-store" products can be just as satisfying as department store products. One of the two emails was from a fella who (and forgive me if I'm wrong) had the "barefoot and pregnant" mentality.

We won't go there.

Recently a woman said to me, "I have tried to figure out how you manage all the balls you juggle . . . and I have decided you take care of yourself. You have inspired me to do the same."

I hope this book has inspired you to take care of yourself physically, but more importantly I hope it has inspired you to give time over to the care of your spiritual self. I hope you've been stirred to be the most beautiful bride for the most wonderful of Bridegrooms!

> Charm is deceptive, and beauty is fleeting;
> but a woman who fears the LORD is to be praised.
>
> Proverbs 31:30

NOTES

Chapter 3: Naptime, Bedtime, and Time Away

1. Merriam-Webster's online dictionary.

Chapter 4: Spas and Salons

1. NIV Study Bible text on Isaiah 55:1, copyright 1985 by Zondervan.
2. This is a partial list. You may find other walk-in/discount hair salons in your area that are not listed here.

Chapter 5: Massage

1. www.mamashealth.com/massage/sweed.asp

Chapter 6: Skin Protection

1. www.skincancer.org/artificial/index.php
2. Author's note: if you suspect that you have any type of skin cancer, please consult your physician immediately.
3. bible.crosswalk.com/Commentaries/GillsExpositionoftheBible/

Chapter 7: Skin Exfoliation

1. Music and lyrics by Elisha A. Hoffman.

Chapter 9: The Face

1. As a side note from the author, a portion of the royalties from this work has gone to a ministry that feeds children in third world countries.
2. www.houstonfaces.com/wrinkles_lines.html

Chapter 10: Eyes, the Window to the Soul

1. Charles Haddon Spurgeon, *The Treasury of David* (Nashville: Thomas Nelson, 1997), 887.

2. Lisa Kasanicky, "Combating Dark Eye Circles," www.azcentral.com/style/articles/0702darkcircles.html, July 2, 2003.

Chapter 11: The Old Kisser

1. The product I'm referencing is from the Lancome line, Rouge Absolu Crème.

Chapter 12: Hands and Feet

1. CLASS is an acronym for Christian Leaders Authors Speakers Seminar. For more information, go to www.CLASServices.com

2. Taken from The NAS New Testament Greek Lexicon (Strong's Number 3741), bible.crosswalk.com/Lexicons/Greek/grk.cgi?number=3741&version=nas

3. Information taken from beauty.indobase.com/nail-care/

Chapter 13: Fragrance

1. Taken in part from ask.yahoo.com/20030226.html

Chapter 14: Fashion

1. Gale Hayman, *How Do I Look?* (New York: Random House, 1996), xiii.

2. bible.crosswalk.com/Lexicons/NewTestamentGreek/ and bible.crosswalk.com/Lexicons/OldTestamentHebrew/

Eva Marie Everson is an award-winning author, a successful speaker, and a radio personality. She has also led numerous Bible studies and women's retreats and is the coauthor of *The Potluck Club* and *The Potluck Club—Trouble's Brewing*. She lives in Central Florida.

Good friends, great food.

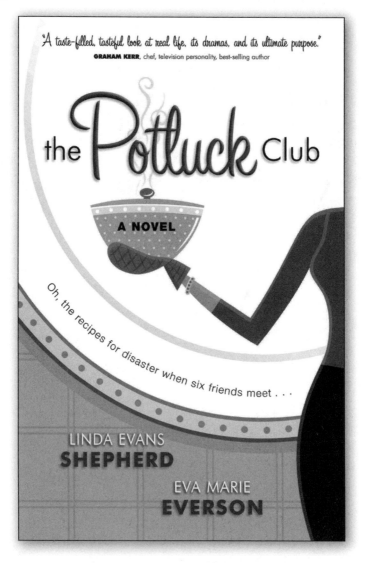

"A taste-filled, tasteful look at real life, its dramas, and its ultimate purpose."
GRAHAM KERR, chef, television personality, best-selling author

the **Potluck** Club

A NOVEL

Oh, the recipes for disaster when six friends meet . . .

LINDA EVANS
SHEPHERD

EVA MARIE
EVERSON

Don't miss the first two installments of

and a pinch of prayer!

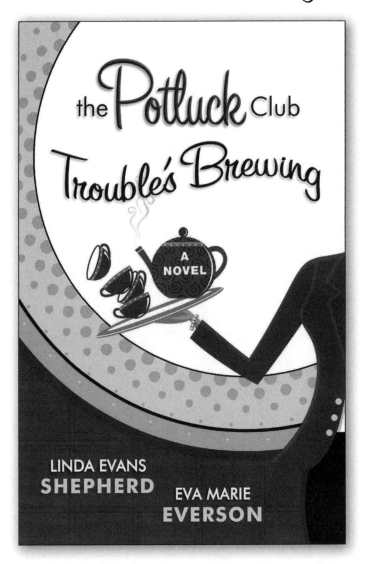

the **Potluck** Club

Trouble's Brewing

A NOVEL

LINDA EVANS
SHEPHERD

EVA MARIE
EVERSON

The Potluck Club's savory adventures

℞ Revell
www.revellbooks.com